Diabetes in Pregnancy

Lisa E. Moore
Editor

Diabetes in Pregnancy

The Complete Guide to
Management

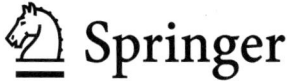 Springer

Editor
Lisa E. Moore
Texas Tech Health Sciences Center
Paul L. Foster School of Medicine
El Paso, TX
USA

ISBN 978-3-319-65517-8   ISBN 978-3-319-65518-5   (eBook)
https://doi.org/10.1007/978-3-319-65518-5

Library of Congress Control Number: 2017963057

Printed on acid-free paper

This Springer imprint is published by Springer Nature
The registered company is Springer International Publishing AG
The registered company address is: Gewerbestrasse 11, 6330 Cham, Switzerland

Contents

About the Editor

Dr. Lisa Moore is professor and chief of the division of maternal–fetal medicine at the Paul L Foster School of Medicine at Texas Tech Health Sciences center in El Paso, Texas. She is also the director of the diabetes in pregnancy program and has ongoing research in the medical management of diabetes in pregnancy. She received her medical degree from Duke University medical school followed by a residency in obstetrics and gynecology at the Medical College of Georgia and Fellowship in Maternal–Fetal medicine at the University of Mississippi.

List of Contributors

Sushila Arya, MD, FACOG Department of Obstetrics and Gynecology, Paul L. Foster School of Medicine, Texas Tech University Health Sciences Center El Paso, El Paso, TX, USA

Diana Clokey, MSRD, RPH, CDE Albuquerque, NM, USA

Sanja Kupesic, MD, PhD Department of Obstetrics and Gynecology, Paul L. Foster School of Medicine, Texas Tech University Health Sciences Center El Paso, El Paso, TX, USA

Carla Ann Martinez, MD Division of Maternal Fetal Medicine, Department of Obstetrics and Gynecology, Texas Tech University Health Sciences Center El Paso Paul L. Foster School of Medicine, El Paso, TX, USA

Lisa E. Moore, MD, FACOG Department of Obstetrics and Gynecology, Texas Tech University Health Sciences Center El Paso, Paul L. Foster School of Medicine, El Paso, TX, USA

Ellen Mozurkewich, MD, MS Obstetrics and Gynecology, University of New Mexico, MSC 10 5580, 1 University of New Mexico, Albuquerque, NM, USA

Valerie Rappaport, MD Division of Maternal Fetal Medicine, Department of Obstetrics and Gynecology, University of New Mexico Health Sciences Center, Albuquerque, NM, USA

Chapter 1
Pathophysiology of Insulin Resistance

Lisa E. Moore

Fast Facts

- All women have a 50–60% decrease in insulin sensitivity as the pregnancy progresses. Women who develop gestational diabetes have preexisting glucose intolerance upon which this normal pregnancy effect is superimposed.
- Increased insulin resistance helps with glucose transfer to the fetus.
- The placentas of women with gestational diabetes are larger in both size and weight and histologically demonstrate ischemic changes, immature villi, and fibrinoid necrosis of villi.

L.E. Moore, MD, FACOG
Department of Obstetrics and Gynecology,
Texas Tech University Health Sciences Center El Paso,
Paul L. Foster School of Medicine, El Paso, TX, USA
e-mail: lisa.e.moore@ttuhsc.edu

© Springer International Publishing AG 2018   1
L.E. Moore (ed.), *Diabetes in Pregnancy*,
https://doi.org/10.1007/978-3-319-65518-5_1

1.1 Introduction

The World Health Organization (WHO) classifies diabetes as DM type 1 characterized by autoimmune destruction of the beta cells of the pancreas, DM type 2 characterized by insulin resistance and relative insulin insufficiency, gestational diabetes (GDM) which is carbohydrate intolerance identified during pregnancy and is also characterized by insulin resistance and relative insulin insufficiency, and rare types of diabetes such as drug-induced diabetes or abnormalities of beta cell function. Gestational diabetes and type 2 diabetes are generally considered to be the same disease manifesting at different times in life. The pregnancy is believed to unmask the tendency toward type 2 diabetes, and it should be noted that the 5-year risk of developing type 2 diabetes in women with GDM is as high as 60% [1].

To understand how gestational diabetes develops, it is necessary first to understand when and how glucose is used by maternal-fetal-placental unit.

Glucose and amino acids are the primary nutrients for the developing fetus. During human pregnancy, several metabolic changes occur to promote efficient glucose transport, from the mother, across the placenta, to the developing conceptus. It is likely that during human evolution, these changes were effective and not harmful. When this physiologic process interacts with the modern lifestyle with a carbohydrate-rich diet and an obesity epidemic, gestational diabetes is the result.

1.2 Insulin Resistance

Insulin release from beta cells is stimulated by the presence of high glucose levels in the blood. Insulin then stimulates the entry of that glucose into muscle cells and adipose cells as well as other types of tissues. As blood glucose levels fall, insulin secretion also decreases or stops. The action of insulin is mediated by the insulin receptor which is found in the plasma membrane. The insulin receptor is made up of two alpha subunits, which are extracellular and contain the domains that bind to insulin, and two beta subunits in the cytoplasm. When insulin binds to the alpha subunits, the tyrosine residues in the beta subunit are given a phosphate group (tyrosine phosphorylation) which activates the receptor.

The activated receptor then phosphorylates certain intracellular proteins called insulin receptor substrates (IRS-1 to IRS-6).

In skeletal muscle, phosphorylation of IRS-1 activates the phosphatidylinositol 3-kinase (PI 3-kinase). PI 3-kinase ultimately triggers translocation of the glucose transporter.

Glucose enters cells by facilitated diffusion via a glucose transporter. Glucose transporter 4 (GLUT4) is the most abundant glucose transporter in skeletal muscle. Normally the transporters are "stored" in cytoplasmic vesicles when not in use. Activation of the insulin receptor substrates as described above causes the vesicles containing the glucose transporters to fuse to the membrane allowing the glucose transporter to be inserted into the membrane which allows the cell to use glucose.

Studies have demonstrated that patients with GDM have less phosphorylation of the insulin receptor than women with normal glucose tolerance. The amount of IRS-1 protein is decreased in the skeletal muscle of obese pregnant women and women with GDM by 30–50% [2].

1.3   The Role of the Placenta

Glucose and amino acids are the primary nutrients for the fetus. The placenta serves as the interface between the maternal circulation and the fetal circulation. This becomes important because (1) several placental-derived hormones are believed to play a role in insulin resistance and (2) the transport of nutrients across the placenta contributes to the fetopathy of diabetes.

The syncytiotrophoblasts have two polarized membranes: one on the maternal side consisting of microvilli and one on the fetal side which is mostly a basal plasma membrane.

Glucose crosses the placenta by facilitated diffusion. The main transporter in the placenta is glucose transporter 1 (GLUT1). GLUT1 is asymmetrically distributed in the placenta with a higher concentration on the maternal side in the microvilli and a significantly lower concentration on the fetal side [3, 4]. GLUT1 function does not depend on the presence of insulin. However, in patients with GDM, higher levels of GLUT1 on the fetal side have been reported which may translate into higher levels of glucose in the fetus.

In a study of women given radiolabeled glucose before delivery, it was demonstrated that 95% of fetal blood glucose is derived from maternal blood glucose [5]. Glucose transfer from mother to fetus is facilitated by a transporter but also requires a concentration gradient. On average, fetal blood glucose is about 15 mg/dL less than maternal blood glucose.

Insulin and large protein hormones do not cross the placenta, and insulin has limited if any role in placental uptake of glucose because the placenta does not express GLUT4 transporters.

The following placental-derived hormones have been implicated in the development of insulin resistance:

Progesterone is known to enhance insulin release from the pancreas.

Cortisol increases during pregnancy to 3× the nonpregnant value. High cortisol increases insulin resistance in the skeletal muscle and increases hepatic glucose production.

Leptin increases during second and third trimester, plays a role in satiety and obesity, and is elevated in women with GDM.

Adiponectin is a protein made in adipocytes; low levels are associated with GDM and type 2 diabetes.

Human placental growth hormone (hPGH) is similar to human growth hormone (13 different amino acids) which increases up to 8× during pregnancy and is shown to cause severe insulin resistance in transgenic mice. hPGH interferes with the PI 3-kinase pathway.

Human placental lactogen rises almost tenfold during pregnancy. HPL stimulates the release of fatty acids and lipids from fat cells. HPL is elevated when blood glucose is low and decreased when blood glucose is high. HPL causes the pancreas to release insulin.

Tumor necrosis factor-α (TNF-α) is a cytokine. Infusion in rats and incubation with the human skeletal muscle induce insulin resistance. It has been shown to reduce insulin receptor tyrosine kinase activity.

1.4   Summary

The development of insulin resistance in pregnancy allows a steady supply of glucose to the fetus. The pathophysiology of insulin resistance is multifactorial and includes decreased expression of the insulin receptor (IR), decreased phosphorylation of the insulin receptor, and decreased insulin receptor substrate (IRS-1) which causes decreased PI 3-kinase leading to decreased number of glucose transporters. Pregnancy hormones also play a significant role.

References

1. Poulakos P, Mintziori G, Tsirou E, Taousani E, Savvaki D, Harizopoulou V, Goulis DG. Comments on gestational diabetes mellitus: from pathophysiology to clinical practice. Hormones. 2015;14(3):335–44. doi:10.14310/horm.2002.1570.
2. Barbour LA, McCurdy CE, Hernandez TL, Kirwan JP, Catalano PM, Friedman JE. Cellular mechanisms for insulin resistance in normal pregnancy and gestational diabetes. Diabetes Care. 2007;30(Suppl 2):S112–9. doi:10.2337/dc07-s202.
3. Larque E, Ruiz-Palacios M, Koletzko B. Placental regulation of fetal nutrient supply. Curr Opin Clin Nutr Metab Care. 2013;16(3):292–7. doi:10.1097/MCO.0b013e32835e3674.
4. Lager S, Powell TL. Regulation of nutrient transport across the placenta. J Pregnancy. 2012;2012:179827. doi:10.1155/2012/179827.
5. Staat BC, Galan HL, Harwood JE, Lee G, Marconi AM, Paolini CL, Cheung A, Battaglia FC. Transplacental supply of mannose and inositol in uncomplicated pregnancies using stable isotopes. J Clin Endocrinol Metab. 2012;97(7):2497–502. doi:10.1210/jc.2011-1800.

Chapter 2
Fetal and Neonatal Consequences of Maternal Diabetes

Lisa E. Moore

Fast Facts

- In the 1950s, Pederson from the University of Copenhagen theorized that excessive maternal glucose crossed the placenta causing fetal hyperinsulinemia and macrosomia (the Pederson hypothesis).
- In the 1980s, Freinkel from Northwestern University presented a lecture theorizing that alterations in metabolic states could function as a teratogen.
- Recent studies have focused on pregnancy as a critical period during which the developing fetus is programmed with an increased risk for noncommunicable diseases such as obesity, diabetes, and heart disease.

L.E. Moore, MD, FACOG
Department of Obstetrics and Gynecology,
Texas Tech University Health Sciences Center El Paso,
Paul L. Foster School of Medicine, El Paso, TX, USA
e-mail: lisa.e.moore@ttuhsc.edu

© Springer International Publishing AG 2018
L.E. Moore (ed.), *Diabetes in Pregnancy*,
https://doi.org/10.1007/978-3-319-65518-5_2

2.1   Diabetic Embryopathy

High concentrations of glucose are a known teratogen. It has been estimated that each year 800 babies are born in the United States with diabetes-associated anomalies. Diabetes-related anomalies occur in all organ systems; however, the most commonly affected systems are the heart, the genitourinary, the craniofacial, and the brain and spine. Uncontrolled blood glucose during the first 7 weeks of pregnancy is the concerning period. The risk of an anomaly increases linearly with the amount of maternal hyperglycemia during that crucial time.

2.1.1   Yolk Sac Theory

The yolk sac is the first vascular system to develop during embryogenesis. It contains the vitelline circulation which provides nutrients to the embryo and also produces erythrocytes. Exposure of mouse embryos to high glucose levels causes anomalies in a variety of disparate organ systems and can cause death. In mice, yolk sac angiogenesis is disrupted so that some embryos show no development of vasculature and others have vasculature with no branching or lack of distinction between arteries and veins [1].

In humans, under high levels of glucose, yolk sac capillaries and vitelline vessels are sparse, and cells in the yolk sac have reduced numbers of ribosomes and mitochondria.

Two pathways appear to operate to cause these effects. Hypoxia-inducible factor 1 (HIF-1) is, as its name implies, an oxygen-sensitive protein that controls the expression of angiogenic growth factors. Normally, reduced oxygen levels allow HIF-1 to accumulate in the embryo which then initiates transcription of angiogenic factors. Hyperglycemia reduces the amount of HIF-1. Knockout mice for HIF-1 develop vascular anomalies similar to those seen in mice embryos exposed to hyperglycemia.

Vascular endothelial growth factor (VEGF) is a protein produced by cells that initiates angiogenesis. VEGF is down-regulated in the setting of hyperglycemia.

2.1.2   Oxygen Free Radicals

High glucose levels interrupt electron transport in the mitochondria causing free oxygen radicals. Hyperglycemia also reduces antioxidants in the cells. Treating embryos cultured in a hyperglycemic environment with antioxidants decreases the rate of malformations. Table 2.1 is a list of common fetal anomalies associated with poorly controlled diabetes.

2.2   Neonatal Complications of Diabetes

2.2.1   Lung Function (RDS)

Respiratory distress syndrome (RDS) also called hyaline membrane disease occurs when the alveoli are not able to remain open due to either a lack of or an insufficient amount of surfactant. Signs and symptoms of RDS include tachypnea, nasal flaring or retractions, radiographic evidence of hyaline membrane disease, and/or persistent oxygen requirement. Babies of diabetic mothers may develop RDS even if they are not premature. Neonatal hyperinsulinemia due to high levels of blood glucose has been shown to interfere with the incorporation of choline into lecithin.

Pregnancies with good glycemic control have no increased risk of RDS.

2.2.2   Macrosomia

Macrosomia is an estimated fetal weight greater than 4500 g. Up to 50% of patients with GDM and 40% of patients with

TABLE 2.1 Common fetal anomalies associated with diabetes

Heart	Brain and spine	Genitourinary	Craniofacial	Skeletal
Hypoplastic heart	Anencephaly	Renal agenesis	Cleft lip	Syringomyelia
Atrial septal defect	Holoprosencephaly		Cleft palate	Sacral agenesis
Ventricular septal defect	Encephalocele		Microtia	Vertebral defects
Double outlet transposition	Hydrocephaly		Eye defects	Limb defects
Tetralogy of Fallot	Microcephaly		Micrognathia	
	Spina bifida			
	Coarctation			

preexisting diabetes have macrosomic neonates. Infants of diabetic mothers disproportionately accumulate fat in the shoulders and chest increasing the risk of shoulder dystocia. National statistics indicate that only 1.5% of newborns in the United States weigh more than 4500 g.

Large for gestational age (LGA) is defined as a birth weight equal to or greater than the 90th percentile for a given gestational age.

2.2.3 Hypoglycemia

Neonatal hypoglycemia is a blood glucose <40 mg/dL in the first 12 h of life. Persistent maternal hyperglycemia results in the fetus having high blood glucose (fetal levels are only 15 mg/dL on average less than maternal levels). The fetal pancreas increases its insulin production and may have beta cell hyperplasia in response. When the umbilical cord is cut, that high level of glucose is abruptly stopped, but the fetal pancreas continues its high output. Maternal normoglycemia in the 6 h immediately preceding delivery can decrease the risk of neonatal hypoglycemia.

2.2.4 Hypocalcemia

Neonatal hypocalcemia is an ionized calcium <4 mg/dL or a total serum calcium <7 mg/dL. Most neonates are asymptomatic and the condition resolves without treatment. Screening for hypocalcemia is recommended only when symptoms such as lethargy, apnea, seizures, or jitteriness are present.

2.2.5 Hyperbilirubinemia

Neonatal hyperbilirubinemia (neonatal jaundice) is caused by the breakdown of fetal hemoglobin which the neonatal liver is unable to manage efficiently.

2.2.6 Shoulder Dystocia

Shoulder dystocia is defined as delivery of the fetal head with impedance of delivery of the fetal shoulders. When birth weight is greater than 4500 g, the risk of shoulder dystocia is between 9.2 and 24%. When the mother is diabetic and the birth weight is greater than 4500 g, the risk increases to 19–50%. Consequences of shoulder dystocia include clavicular fracture and brachial plexus injury.

2.2.7 Stillbirth

Intrauterine death is the most feared of all complications of diabetes. Type 1 diabetes confers a three- to fivefold increase in the risk of stillbirth. In women with type 2 diabetes, the risk is increased though the amount of increase varies with populations. In some studies, the risk of stillbirth in type 2 diabetes is higher than the risk of type 1. It is theorized that this may be due to underdiagnosis or undertreatment. In women with GDM, some studies have found an increased risk, and other studies have found no increased risk of stillbirth. The common theme is that in the setting of poor glycemic control, regardless of the type of diabetes, the risk of stillbirth is increased.

2.3   In Utero Programming

It has been known since the early twentieth century that pregnancies complicated by diabetes produce babies with a high birth weight. However, the long-term consequences of exposure to diabetes in utero are only now being appreciated. Large epidemiologic studies indicate that there is an increased risk of diabetes, metabolic syndrome, obesity, and cardiovascular disease in the offspring of pregnancies complicated by diabetes.

Epigenetics is the term for changes in gene expression that can be transmitted to offspring that do not involve changes in

DNA sequences. Epigenetic mechanisms include DNA methylation, noncoding RNAs, and histone changes. Addition of a methyl group to DNA (DNA methylation), for instance, can cause transcriptional silencing of genes.

There are some very interesting human studies of epigenetics. The "Dutch Hunger Winter" was a famine in 1944–1945 in the German-occupied Netherlands. Adults who were conceived during that time (60 years earlier) were compared to their same gender siblings. DNA methylation was 5.2% less in the patients conceived during the famine [2].

A study of DNA methylation in the placenta and cord blood showed that maternal blood glucose was associated with the amount of methylation of the adiponectin gene in the placenta. On the maternal side of the placenta, lower levels of methylation correlated with increased insulin resistance. On the fetal side, lower amounts of methylation were associated with higher maternal blood glucose [3].

2.3.1 Obesity

In 1983 the Pima Indians of Arizona were found to have a very high rate of obesity in children whose mothers had diabetes. Fifty-eight percent of those children weighed more than one hundred and forty percent of their ideal body weight between the ages of 15 and 19 [4].

A study from Kaiser Permanente investigated 9439 mother-child pairs. The study found that increasing levels of blood glucose during pregnancy were associated with an increased risk of obesity at age 5–7 in the children. They also suggested that fasting hyperglycemia was an important predictor of future childhood obesity [5].

2.3.2 Type 2 Diabetes

The SEARCH case-control study looked at 79 adolescents (<20 years) with type 2 diabetes and 190 controls who were not diabetic [6]. The population was multiethnic: Hispanic, African-American, and non-Hispanic white. 30.4% of youth with type 2 DM were exposed in utero to maternal diabetes, and 57% had in utero exposure to maternal obesity.

2.3.3 Neurological and Psychological Development

Several studies since the early 1990s have shown an association between maternal altered metabolic states and changes in the neurologic and psychological well-being in the offspring.

A population-based study of singletons exposed to gestational diabetes compared to unexposed singletons looked at hospitalization for neuropsychiatric disease. The study found that gestational diabetes was an independent risk factor for long-term neuropsychiatric morbidity in the offspring. They also demonstrated that children exposed to GDM developed neuropsychiatric disease at a younger age than unexposed children [7].

Researchers from Johns Hopkins School of Public Health found that the combination of gestational diabetes and maternal obesity was associated with an increased risk of autism spectrum disorder and intellectual disability in the offspring [8].

2.3.4 Cardiovascular Disease

Studies of the fetal origin of cardiovascular disease show a high correlation with fetal undergrowth. However, there is evidence that fetal overgrowth or macrosomia is associated with an increased risk of elevated systolic blood pressure. A meta-analysis of the available data demonstrated that in utero exposure to maternal diabetes was associated with increased systolic blood pressure during childhood in male offspring [9].

2.4   Summary

Pregestational uncontrolled diabetes is associated with congenital anomalies which may affect several organ systems. After organogenesis, fetal and neonatal effects include macrosomia, hypoglycemia, and respiratory distress syndrome.

Exposure to maternal diabetes and obesity in utero may confer a lifetime risk of obesity, metabolic syndrome, diabetes, and cardiovascular disease to the offspring. There is also evolving literature indicating an associated risk of neuropsychiatric disease.

References

1. Dong D, Reece EA, Lin X, Wu Y, Arias Villela N, Yang P. New development of the yolk sac theory in diabetic embryopathy: molecular mechanism and link to structural birth defects. Am J Obstet Gynecol. 2016;214(2):192–202. doi:10.1016/j.ajog.2015.09.082.
2. Heijmans BT, Tobi EW, Stein AD, Putter H, Blauw GJ, Susser ES, Slagboom PE, Lumey LH. Persistent epigenetic differences associated with prenatal exposure to famine in humans. Proc Natl Acad Sci U S A. 2008;105(44):17046–9. doi:10.1073/pnas.0806560105.
3. Bouchard L, Hivert MF, Guay SP, St-Pierre J, Perron P, Brisson D. Placental adiponectin gene DNA methylation levels are associated with mothers' blood glucose concentration. Diabetes. 2012;61(5):1272–80. doi:10.2337/db11-1160.
4. Pettitt DJ, Baird HR, Aleck KA, Bennett PH, Knowler WC. Excessive obesity in offspring of Pima Indian women with diabetes during pregnancy. N Engl J Med. 1983;308(5):242–5. doi:10.1056/NEJM198302033080502.
5. Hillier TA, Pedula KL, Schmidt MM, Mullen JA, Charles MA, Pettitt DJ. Childhood obesity and metabolic imprinting: the ongoing effects of maternal hyperglycemia. Diabetes Care. 2007;30(9):2287–92. doi:10.2337/dc06-2361.
6. Dabelea D, Mayer-Davis EJ, Lamichhane AP, D'Agostino RB Jr, Liese AD, Vehik KS, Narayan KM, Zeitler P, Hamman RF.

Association of intrauterine exposure to maternal diabetes and obesity with type 2 diabetes in youth: the SEARCH case-control study. Diabetes Care. 2008;31(7):1422–6. doi:10.2337/dc07-2417.

7. Nahum Sacks K, Friger M, Shoham-Vardi I, Abokaf H, Spiegel E, Sergienko R, Landau D, Sheiner E. Prenatal exposure to gestational diabetes mellitus as an independent risk factor for long-term neuropsychiatric morbidity of the offspring. Am J Obstet Gynecol. 2016;215:380.e1–7. doi:10.1016/j.ajog.2016.03.030.

8. Li M, Fallin MD, Riley A, Landa R, Walker SO, Silverstein M, Caruso D, Pearson C, Kiang S, Dahm JL, Hong X, Wang G, Wang MC, Zuckerman B, Wang X. The association of maternal obesity and diabetes with autism and other developmental disabilities. Pediatrics. 2016;137(2):e20152206. doi:10.1542/peds.2015-2206.

9. Aceti A, Santhakumaran S, Logan KM, Philipps LH, Prior E, Gale C, Hyde MJ, Modi N. The diabetic pregnancy and offspring blood pressure in childhood: a systematic review and meta-analysis. Diabetologia. 2012;55(11):3114–27. doi:10.1007/s00125-012-2689-8.

Chapter 3
Preconception Counseling

Lisa E. Moore

Fast Facts

- The preconception visit represents an opportunity to affect lifestyle change at a time when the patient is most motivated.
- Contraceptive counseling is an important aspect of the care of women with diabetes.

3.1 Introduction

Poorly controlled type 1 or type 2 diabetes during pregnancy is associated with an increased risk of a congenital fetal anomaly, increased risk of fetal death, risk of fetal macrosomia, risk of admission to the neonatal intensive care unit, and risk of neonatal hypoglycemia. Maternal end-organ damage may progress during pregnancy, and diabetes is associated with an increased risk of hypertensive disease of pregnancy.

L.E. Moore, MD, FACOG
Department of Obstetrics and Gynecology, Texas Tech University Health Sciences Center El Paso, Paul L. Foster School of Medicine, El Paso, TX, USA
e-mail: lisa.e.moore@ttuhsc.edu

© Springer International Publishing AG 2018
L.E. Moore (ed.), *Diabetes in Pregnancy*,
https://doi.org/10.1007/978-3-319-65518-5_3

17

The goal of preconception counseling is to inform patients of these risks, to provide guidance on ways to reduce or eliminate these risks, and, most importantly, to provide support in achieving any necessary lifestyle modifications to optimize the outcome of a pregnancy.

3.1.1 Preconception Evaluation

The preconception evaluation and counseling should be done in two separate visits. Ideally, patients who are not meeting glycemic goals or with significant comorbidities should present at least 6 months prior to attempting pregnancy. This will allow time to normalize blood glucose, to make appropriate changes to medications, and to optimize other disease processes.

During the first visit, a complete physical examination and laboratory evaluation should be performed which include the following:

- Screen for tobacco or other substance use and provide counseling as needed.
- Screen patients for sexually transmitted infections.
- Update vaccinations (Tdap, MMR, influenza, Hep B, varicella) as needed.
- Foot examination for nonhealing wounds.
- Cardiac auscultation, peripheral pulses, and an EKG.
- 24 h urine collection for protein and creatinine clearance.
- Complete metabolic panel.
- Hemoglobin A1C (HA1C)—the A1C is the best indicator of glycemic control, and when elevated during organogenesis, there is a significant risk of fetal anomaly.
- TSH—to evaluate thyroid function and treat as indicated.
- Eye exam—refer patient for a dilated eye exam to rule out retinopathy if not done in the last year.

The patient can be scheduled to return in 1–2 weeks when the laboratory results are available. Counseling should be culturally appropriate and individualized based on lab results, physical examination, and known comorbidities. At that second visit, goals should be set such as weight loss or to normalize the A1C. Physician support for these goals can include scheduled visits, nutrition counseling, and referrals to a dietician or an exercise program. Referrals can also be made to other specialists as indicated.

3.1.2   Pregnancy Planning and Contraception

Women with diabetes should use contraception. The choice of contraception can be based on individual preference with consideration of each patient's needs and history. The offering of effective contraception should be considered part of the management of diabetes in women. This is particularly true of adolescents. In patients who desire a pregnancy, contraception should be continued until blood glucose is adequately controlled and comorbidities are managed.

3.1.3   Target Blood Glucose and HA1C

Hyperglycemia is the primary culprit in the risks associated with diabetes in pregnancy. Studies consistently demonstrate that tight glycemic control prior to pregnancy, during the period of organogenesis, and continuing through the pregnancy is associated with improved outcomes.

The HA1C should be below 6.5%. This level has been shown to reduce the risk of congenital anomalies.

Daily self-monitoring of blood glucose can be an aid to achieving the desired reduction in A1C.

Preconceptually, a fasting blood glucose between 80 and 110 mg/dL and a 2 h postprandial blood glucose of <155 mg/dL is the goal. These levels will achieve a HA1C <6.5%.

3.1.4   Folic Acid Supplementation

Women with diabetes have a higher than baseline risk of neural tube defects. The American Diabetes Association recommends supplementation with 600 mcg/day of folic acid [1].

3.1.5   Weight Loss

Diet, exercise, and weight loss are the holy trinity of diabetes management for patients with type 2 diabetes. Referral for dietary counseling and initiation of an exercise plan will benefit women in need of those services. Weight loss will improve glycemic control and will decrease the risk of obesity-associated complications such as cesarean delivery.

3.1.6   Bariatric Surgery

Bariatric surgery is considered an appropriate treatment for people with type 2 diabetes and obesity who are unable to achieve treatment targets with diet, exercise, and medical therapy [2, 3].

Pregnancy following bariatric surgery is considered safe. It is recommended to wait 1 to 2 years after surgery before attempting pregnancy. Pregnancy may increase the risk of certain complications depending on the specific procedure. Bariatric surgery may decrease the ability to absorb certain nutrients which may require supplementation during pregnancy.

3.1.7   Management of Comorbidities/Medications

Glycemic control—currently the only oral agents which have been well studied during pregnancy are metformin, glyburide, and acarbose. Metformin and glyburide are supported for use by ACOG. Patients on these medications can usually continue them. Other oral agents should be discontinued. Insulin is still considered the goal standard. Women on the insulin pump can continue on the pump through pregnancy.

Women with type1 or type 2 diabetes often have chronic hypertension and/or hyperlipidemia. Statins are contraindicated in pregnancy. Data regarding the absolute risk is conflicting. It is recommended to discontinue statins in women planning to become pregnant or as soon a pregnancy is discovered.

Women with chronic hypertension are often placed on angiotensin converting enzyme inhibitors (ACEI) or angiotensin receptor blockers (ARBs) due to their renal protective effect. These should be discontinued and another type of antihypertensive initiated in women who are planning a pregnancy. Options include labetolol, methyldopa, or a calcium channel blocker such as Plendil or nifedipine.

Hypo-/hyperthyroidism—achieving euthyroid status improves pregnancy outcomes and may improve the chance of conceiving.

Renal dysfunction—patients with renal dysfunction should be comanaged with a nephrologist if possible.

3.1.8 Risks to the Fetus and Neonate

Diabetic embryopathy—elevated blood glucose is a teratogen. The risk of a fetal anomaly is increased two to four times in women with uncontrolled blood glucose. This may include malformations in various organ systems though cardiac and central nervous system defects are most common.

Macrosomia—macrosomia is defined as fetal birth weight >4000 g. Large babies are at risk for birth trauma such as a broken clavicle or injury to the brachial plexus. During vaginal delivery, there is, in addition to the fetal risk, the maternal risk of pelvic damage resulting in fistula development or varying degrees of incontinence.

Fetal demise—the risk of fetal death is increased in women with diabetes and has been shown to increase with increasing HA1C. In the setting of strict glycemic control, the risk of fetal death is not different than the baseline risk seen in nondiabetics.

Medical complications/admission to the NICU—babies of diabetic mothers with poor control may be unable to maintain blood glucose levels after delivery. This is because the neonatal pancreas has become accustomed to high glucose. Once the connection to the mother is severed, the pancreas continues to secrete insulin resulting in hypoglycemia.

Increased production of red blood cells may occur in large babies due to chronic hypoxia as they have outgrown the placental ability to support the fetal size. Babies may also have hyperbilirubinemia requiring phototherapy due to increased destruction of red blood cells. Hypocalcemia may present as jitteriness or seizures and is believed to be due to delayed synthesis of parathyroid hormone.

Babies of diabetic mothers may also experience growth failure. Though less common, it is most often seen in women with diabetes and associated cardiovascular or renal disease.

Respiratory distress—high levels of glucose interfere with the incorporation of choline into the surfactant molecule. Babies may present shortly after birth with tachypnea, retractions, and nasal flaring.

Epigenetic programming—there is convincing evidence that exposure to high levels of blood glucose during pregnancy may predispose the fetus to childhood obesity and early development of type 2 diabetes.

3.1.9   Risks to the Patient

Diabetic ketoacidosis (DKA)—patients with type 1 diabetes experience a lowered threshold for DKA. Morning sickness can exacerbate anorexia. During episodes of DKA, there is a significant risk of fetal death.

Renal disease—women with chronic hypertension or impaired kidney function may experience worsening of disease during pregnancy. Women with a serum creatinine >3 mg/dL or a creatinine clearance <50 cm^3/min may experience a permanent decline in renal function during pregnancy [ADA].

Retinopathy—most women with retinopathy will not have worsening of the disease during pregnancy. An exception to this is women with proliferative retinopathy which should be treated prior to pregnancy. Visual changes due to proliferative retinopathy may be permanent.

Cardiovascular disease—there is an increased risk of macro- and microvascular disease. The magnitude of the risk is increased with comorbidities such as hypertension or renal disease.

Hypertensive disorders of pregnancy—the risk of pre-eclampsia and gestational hypertension is increased three- to fourfold in patients with diabetes.

3.2   Summary

The risk of a poor pregnancy outcome is increased in women with pre-gestational diabetes. Preconception counseling provides an opportunity to inform patients of the risk of diabetes in pregnancy and to use that time when the patient is most motivated to initiate lifestyle changes that will improve both pregnancy outcome and the patient's long-term health status.

References

1. Kitzmiller JL, Block JM, Brown FM, Catalano PM, Conway DL, Coustan DR, Gunderson EP, Herman WH, Hoffman LD, Inturrisi M, Jovanovic LB, Kjos SI, Knopp RH, Montoro MN, Ogata ES, Paramsothy P, Reader DM, Rosenn BM, Thomas AM, Kirkman MS. Managing preexisting diabetes for pregnancy: summary of evidence and consensus recommendations for care. Diabetes Care. 2008;31(5):1060–79. doi:10.2337/dc08-9020.
2. Dixon JB, Zimmet P, Alberti KG, Rubino F. Bariatric surgery: an IDF statement for obese Type 2 diabetes. Obes Res Clin Pract. 2011;5(3):e169–266. doi:10.1016/j.orcp.2011.07.002.
3. Zimmet P, Campbell L, Toomath R, Twigg S, Wittert G, Proietto J. Bariatric surgery to treat severely obese patients with type 2 diabetes: a consensus statement. Obes Res Clin Pract. 2011;5(1):e1–e78. doi:10.1016/j.orcp.2010.11.005.

Chapter 4
Type 1 Diabetes

Lisa E. Moore

> **Fast Facts**
>
> - Being born in the spring is a risk factor for developing type 1 diabetes.
> - Type 1 diabetes is caused by autoimmune destruction of the β-cells of the pancreas.

4.1 Introduction

Type 1 diabetes in pregnancy presents a significant management challenge. Poor glycemic control during organogenesis is the greatest risk factor for diabetes associated fetopathy. Poor control during the pregnancy is associated with a number of adverse outcomes including macrosomia and fetal death. Additionally, pregnancy adds a degree of insulin resistance to an endogenous lack of insulin.

L.E. Moore, MD, FACOG
Department of Obstetrics and Gynecology, Texas Tech University Health Sciences Center El Paso, Paul L. Foster School of Medicine, El Paso, TX, USA
e-mail: lisa.e.moore@ttuhsc.edu

Women with type 1 diabetes can and do have successful pregnancies. Successful management starts before pregnancy and emphasizes strict control of blood glucose throughout.

4.2   Epidemiology

Depending on the population studied, up to 15% of pregnancies are complicated by diabetes. Less than 1% of those patients will have type 1 diabetes. Globally there are several studies looking at the incidence and outcome of type 1 diabetes particularly in children because the onset of type 1 diabetes is usually during childhood. There is a peak in diagnosis between 5 and 7 years of age and near puberty [1].

Greater than 85% of diabetes in persons <20 years of age worldwide is type 1 diabetes. An exception to this is found among the Navajo. In the SEARCH study, the majority of Navajo youth with diabetes had type 2 diabetes [2, 3]. The incidence of type 1 diabetes is increasing, and the largest increase is noted in young children aged 0–4 years [4]. Type 1 diabetes has been diagnosed at all ages. Approximately a fourth of people with type 1 diabetes were diagnosed as adults.

Type 1 diabetes affects males and females equally; however, an interesting pattern has been identified in European population where there is a high incidence of type 1 diabetes. Males are slightly more prevalent than affected females in European high-prevalence populations. In non-European, high-prevalence populations, females predominate.

Other interesting facts are that Finland has the highest rate of type 1 diabetes. Type 1 diabetes is rare in China and India [4].

4.3   Genetics

Multiple haplotypes of the human leukocyte antigen (HLA) region on chromosome 6 have an association with type 1 diabetes. Class I major histocompatibility complex (MHC) genes are associated with increased risk of developing type 1 diabetes.

Up to 95% of children with type 1 diabetes carry a suscep-tibility haplotype. In contrast, less than 5% of people known to carry a susceptible haplotype actually develop clinical disease.

In the United States, the risk of developing type 1 diabetes is 1 in 300 over a lifetime for the general population but increased to 1 in 20 if there is first-degree relative with type 1 diabetes. Children of mothers with type 1 diabetes have a 2–3% risk, and children of affected fathers have a 7% risk. In monozygotic twinning, both twins have type 1 diabetes in 60% of cases. In dizygotic twins, both are affected only 6–10% of the time. These statistics support the concept of a genetic influence.

Environment interacts with genetics in the development of type 1 diabetes. The environmental factors have yet to be identified.

4.4   Pathophysiology

The concept of type 1 diabetes as an autoimmune disease was introduced by George Eisenbarth in 1986. His model of the development of type 1 diabetes contained six stages: (1) genetic susceptibility, (2) a triggering event, (3) development of autoimmunity, (4) progressive loss of insulin secretion with normal blood glucose, (5) overt diabetes with some residual insulin secretion, and finally (6) complete loss of β-cell func-tion [5].

Type 1 diabetes occurs when the pancreatic β-cells in the islets of Langerhans are destroyed. Prior to complete destruc-tion of the β-cells is a state which is called insulinitis. During insulinitis, CD4+ and CD8+ lymphocytes, macrophages, and β-lymphocytes attack the islets of Langerhans. Insulin deficiency is the eventual result. However, it should be clear from the description that insulin deficiency evolves over time and that it is possible to identify patients in the process of developing type 1 diabetes. The development of antibodies to islet cells may precede the development of type 1 diabetes by months to years [1].

4.5   Diagnosis

The hallmark of type 1 diabetes is insulin deficiency due to destruction of β-cells in the pancreas. Depending on where patients are in the disease, they may retain some endogenous insulin production. Differentiating type 1 diabetes in the early stages from type 2 diabetes presents a diagnostic challenge. It is believed that between 5 and 15% of adults who are given a diagnosis of type 2 diabetes may have type 1 disease [1].

Most patients will enter pregnancy with a diagnosis of type 1 diabetes. Patients who are diagnosed during pregnancy typically present in diabetic ketoacidosis due to the added insulin resistance of the pregnancy.

The classic triad of symptomatology of type 1 diabetes is excessive thirst, excessive urination, and weight loss.

Diagnosis of diabetes is made when one of the following criteria is met [6]:

- ≥126 mg/dL after an 8 h fast OR
- ≥200 mg/dL at 2 h after a 75 g glucose load OR
- A1C ≥ 6.5%

After the diagnosis of diabetes, confirmation of type 1 diabetes is made by measurement of C-peptide levels or the presence of anti-β-cell antibodies.

C-peptide is formed during conversion of proinsulin to insulin. An insulin or C-peptide level below 5 μU/mL (0.6 ng/mL) suggests type 1 DM; a fasting C-peptide level greater than 1 ng/dL in a patient who has had diabetes for more than 1–2 years is suggestive of type 2 (i.e., residual β-cell function). The most important diagnostic feature is the presence of antibodies to β-cells. Common anti-β-cell antibodies are insulin-reactive antibodies (IAA), insulinoma-associated autoantigen 2(IA2A), glutamic acid decarboxylase (GADA), and antibodies to zinc transporter 8 (ZnT8A).

4.6   Management in Pregnancy

In addition to routine prenatal care, patients with type 1 DM should have evaluation for end-organ damage at the first prenatal visit. This includes an EKG, a 24 h urine for protein spillage and creatinine clearance, an ophthalmology examination to rule out retinopathy if she has not been examined within the last year, and a HgbA1C to assess the degree of glycemic control over the last 3 months. Between 18 to 22 weeks, a complete evaluation of fetal anatomy including a complete evaluation of the fetal heart to rule out anomalies should be performed. Antenatal testing should be initiated between 28 and 32 weeks, and patients should have monthly sonographic evaluations of fetal growth after 24 weeks. These recommendations are summarized in Box 1.

Pregnant patients with type 1 diabetes should check their blood glucose levels six to seven times daily: before each meal and either 1 or 2 h after meals. Premeal glucose levels should be <100 mg/dL. One-hour postprandials should be <140 mg/dL, and 2 h postprandials should be <120 mg/dL. Blood glucose should never be below 60 mg/dL (hypoglycemia).

Type 1 diabetics usually are managed using two very important numbers:

- The insulin to carbohydrate ratio—how much insulin to take to cover a certain amount of carbohydrate
- The correction factor—how much 1 unit of insulin will drop the blood glucose level

Patients use both of these numbers to calculate how to dose insulin. For example, a patient checks her blood glucose before eating dinner, and it is 150 mg/dL. She plans to eat a meal with approximately 45 g of carbohydrate. Her insulin to carb ratio is 1:10 and her correction factor is 1:30.

She will use the correction factor to correct her premeal blood glucose. She wants to drop her premeal glucose to 100 mg/dL, so she will take 2 units of insulin (correction factor is 1:30 and she needs to lose 50 mg/dL).

She is planning to eat 45 g of carbohydrate, so according to her correction factor, she needs 1 unit per 10 g of carbohydrate. So she will add 4.5 units of insulin. Her total dose of insulin is 6.5 units prior to this meal. She will then check her blood glucose either 1 or 2 h after the meal to see if she corrected appropriately.

4.6.1   1500/1800 Rule

The 1500/1800 rule provides a quick and dirty estimate of the insulin correction factor. Divide the rule by the total daily dose (TDD) of insulin to estimate the correction factor. For regular insulin, use 1500, and for short-acting insulins, use 1800.

> For example, the patient above takes a total of 50 units of regular insulin per day (this means adding up all her doses in a day) 1500/50 = 30. This indicates that her correction factor with regular insulin is 1:30 which means that 1 unit of regular insulin drops her blood glucose to 30 mg/dL.

4.6.2   450/500 or 2.6 Rule

To calculate the insulin to carb ratio or the carbohydrate factor, use the 450/500 rule or the 2.6 rule.

Method 1: multiply weight in pounds by 2.6, and divide by total daily dose of insulin (all types of insulin).

> Example: the woman in the previous example weighs 180 pounds, and she uses a total daily dose of all insulins of 47 units. 180 × 2.6 = 468/47 = 9.9 or an insulin to carbohydrate ratio of 1:10.

Method 2: Using 450 for regular insulin and 500 for short-acting insulin, divide the rule by the TDD to get the carbohydrate factor.

> Example: The patient takes 50 units of regular insulin per day. 450/50 is equal to a correction of 1:9.

4.7 Diet

The American College of Obstetricians and Gynecologists recommend a diet of 24–35 kcal/kg/day with an emphasis on high-fiber foods. Here is an interesting note—if you look at the recommendation, it appears to say to eat 35 kcal/kg of body weight per day. For a 120-pound woman, that would be over a million calories a day. In the United States, when a label says calories, it actually means kcal. So the calories that we are accustomed to seeing are actually kilocalories. For example, a teaspoon of sugar is labeled as 15 calories, but it's actually 15 kcal. So the recommendation is for 35 cal/kg of body weight per day.

All patients with type 1 diabetes must count carbohydrates. As discussed in an earlier section, this is the only way to achieve euglycemia.

4.8 Insulin Therapy

During pregnancy it is rare to encounter a type 1 diabetic who is not already on insulin. In which case, you should adjust the insulin regimen based on postprandial blood glucose values.

For a patient who does not know their correction factor, a starting place is to assign a correction factor of 1:30 which is equivalent to a I/C ratio of 1:10.

A combination of rapid-acting insulin with meals and an intermediate-acting insulin bolused once or twice a day will provide adequate coverage. An alternate is rapid-acting insulin with a long-acting formulation designed to provide steady insulin without a peak such as glargine or detemir.

Initiation of insulin should be weight based with the recognition that type 1 diabetics can be brittle even in pregnancy.

Remember that a weight-based calculation serves as a starting point only. It is unlikely that the patient will be controlled with the first attempt. Insulin dosing should be adjusted up or down to achieve euglycemia and to prevent hypoglycemia. The patient should be informed that several dose changes may be required to achieve control.

There are several different methods of dosing insulin. The correct method depends on the patient's needs and lifestyle.

To calculate a starting daily dose of insulin, multiply weight in kilograms by 0.3–0.6.

> Example: Patient weighs 160 pounds: $160/2.2 = 72.7$ kg $\times 6 =$ a total daily dose (TDD) of 43 units.

4.8.1   Method 1: Regular Insulin and NPH

This is the now less commonly used method of dividing the dose of insulin so that:

2/3 of the TDD is given before breakfast and 1/3 of TDD is given before supper.

1/3 of the morning dose is regular insulin; 2/3 is NPH. The regular covers breakfast and the NPH covers dinner.

1/2 of the evening dose is regular insulin and ½ is NPH. The regular covers the nighttime snack and the NPH covers morning fasting.

> In our example, the patient had a TDD of 43 units.
> $43/3 = 14.3$—this means that 14 units is the evening dose and 28 units is the morning dose.
> $28/3 = 9.3$ (you can round up or down as appropriate).
> Morning dose = 9 units of regular and 18 units of NPH.
> Evening dose = 7 units of regular and 7 units of NPH.

With this regimen, watch out for nighttime hypoglycemia. A nighttime snack must be eaten. Since insulin is taken in the morning for breakfast and lunch and dinner and if those meals are missed, delayed, or if a smaller amount of food than anticipated is eaten, there is a significant risk of hypoglycemia. This is not a good regimen for patients who are unable to eat at the same time each day.

4.8.2 Method 2: Rapid-Acting Insulin and Intermediate Insulin at Bedtime

A quick and easy way to calculate dosing for this method is to take the TDD and simply divide by 4. Continuing with the TDD from the previous example:

43/4 is roughly 11 units.

Give 11 units of rapid-acting insulin (lispro, aspart, Humalog, Novolog) with each meal.

Give 11 units of intermediate-acting insulin (NPH) at bedtime.

In this regimen, NPH will peak 4–8 h after it is taken and is designed to control the fasting in the morning. The "tail" or prolonged activity of NPH may smooth out blood glucose in the mornings, but by afternoon there is a risk of hyperglycemia. Also watch for nighttime hypoglycemia and reduce the amount if needed.

4.8.3 Method 3: Rapid-Acting Insulin and a Basal Insulin

Use the same calculation as in the previous example to calculate rapid-acting insulin dose with meals. The starting dose of glargine (Lantus) is calculated as 1/3 of the total daily dose in patients already on insulin, or you can use 10 units as a starting dose with the plan to titrate as needed.

> The TDD = 43 units from the previous example.
> TDD/4 = 11 units of rapid-acting insulin before each meal.
> TDD/3 = 14 units of basal insulin.

Fourteen units of glargine can be taken at any time but must be taken at the same time each day (glargine must be given in a second syringe because it should not be mixed with other insulins).

An alternate to glargine is Levemir—starting dose is 10 units or 0.1–0.2 units/kg of body weight. It should also be taken at the same time each day and cannot be mixed with other insulins.

Both glargine and Levemir provide steady peakless insulin levels during the day and in theory more closely mimic normal pancreatic secretion of activity and should provide better glucose control.

4.8.4   To Switch from NPH to Glargine

Once-a-day NPH—dose glargine 1:1.
Twice-a-day NPH—give 80% of the total NPH dose.
Premixed insulin—give 80% of the NPH portion of the premix dose.

4.9   Summary

Type 1 diabetes is the result of destruction of insulin-producing β-cells in the pancreas. The incidence of type 1 is increasing worldwide. It is a multifactorial disease indicating that genetic susceptibility in conjunction with an unidentified environmental trigger is believed to be the cause. The usual age of onset of type 1 diabetes is during childhood, and it can be expected that affected women will participate in childbearing. Currently type 1 diabetes is found in less than 1% of pregnancies. These pregnancies are at significant risk of adverse outcome. Tight control of blood glucose ameliorates the risks.

4.10   Additional Information

Type 1 diabetes TrialNet is a cooperation of 18 clinical centers in 7 countries dedicated to the study, prevention, and treatment of type1 diabetes. It is supported by the National Institute of Health (NIH) as well as the ADA and other major diabetes organizations. TrialNet is a gateway for participation in studies to delay progression of type1 diabetes and ways to delay or prevent the development of type1 diabetes. For more information, go to www.DiabetesTrialNet.org.

Box 1 Prenatal Care in Type 1 Diabetes (in Addition to Routine Prenatal Care)

First visit
Hgb A1C
EKG
24 h urine for protein and creatinine clearance
Ophthalmology exam to rule out retinopathy
Ask about dental concerns
Foot exam
Second and third trimester
Initiate antenatal testing at 28 weeks (NST+AFI or BPP)
Monthly evaluation of growth after 24 weeks
Delivery at 38 weeks

Box 2 Methods for Calculating Insulin Dosage

Method 1: regular insulin + intermediate-acting insulin
TDD (0.66) = total morning dose (MD)
MD(0.33) = regular insulin dose in am
MD (0.66) = NPH dose in am
TDD (0.33) = total evening dose (ED)
ED/2 = evening dose of regular insulin
ED/2 = evening dose of NPH
Method 2: rapid-acting insulin + intermediate-acting insulin
TDD/4 = dose of rapid-acting insulin with each meal
TDD/4 = dose of NPH at bedtime
Method 3: rapid-acting insulin + basal insulin
TDD/4 = dose of rapid-acting insulin with each meal
TDD/3 = dose of basal insulin (or start with 10 units and titrate)

References

1. Atkinson MA, Eisenbarth GS, Michels AW. Type 1 diabetes. Lancet. 2014;383(9911):69–82. doi:10.1016/S0140-6736(13)60591-7.
2. Dabelea D, Hanson RL, Bennett PH, Roumain J, Knowler WC, Pettitt DJ. Increasing prevalence of Type II diabetes in American Indian children. Diabetologia. 1998;41(8):904–10. doi:10.1007/s001250051006.
3. Mayer-Davis EJ, Bell RA, Dabelea D, D'Agostino R Jr, Imperatore G, Lawrence JM, Liu L, Marcovina S, Group SfDiYS. The many faces of diabetes in American youth: type 1 and type 2 diabetes in five race and ethnic populations: the SEARCH for Diabetes in Youth Study. Diabetes Care. 2009;32(Suppl 2):S99–101. doi:10.2337/dc09-S201.
4. Maahs DM, West NA, Lawrence JM, Mayer-Davis EJ. Epidemiology of type 1 diabetes. Endocrinol Metab Clin N Am. 2010;39(3):481–97. doi:10.1016/j.ecl.2010.05.011.
5. Eisenbarth GS. Type I diabetes mellitus. A chronic autoimmune disease. N Engl J Med. 1986;314(21):1360–8. doi:10.1056/NEJM198605223142106.
6. American Diabetes Association. Diagnosis and classification of diabetes mellitus. Diabetes Care. 2010;33(Suppl 1):S62–9. doi:10.2337/dc10-S062.

Chapter 5
Type 2 Diabetes

Lisa E. Moore

Fast Facts

- Being overweight or obese is the greatest risk factor for type 2 diabetes.
- Type 2 diabetes is now considered a global health epidemic.
- Programming for early-onset type 2 diabetes is believed to happen in utero.
- Type 2 diabetes and gestational diabetes are believed to be the same disease.

5.1 Introduction

Type 2 diabetes (T2D) is a metabolic disease characterized by hyperglycemia, insulin resistance, and relative insulin deficiency. According to the World Health Organization (WHO), the prevalence of T2D worldwide has become epidemic.

L.E. Moore, MD, FACOG
Department of Obstetrics and Gynecology, Texas Tech University
Health Sciences Center El Paso, Paul L. Foster School of Medicine,
El Paso, TX, USA
e-mail: lisa.e.moore@ttuhsc.edu

Outside of pregnancy, 90% of patients with diabetes have type 2 diabetes. During pregnancy, uncontrolled T2D is associated with an increased risk of fetal anomalies, fetal macrosomia, and fetal death. Because the prevalence of T2D during the childbearing years has increased, many women may go undiagnosed prior to pregnancy.

A study of women with type 2 diabetes during pregnancy found an 11-fold increased risk of congenital anomalies and twofold increased risk of stillbirth in comparison to the general population [1].

5.2   Epidemiology

Worldwide 6.4% of the population had T2D in 2010. Until the latter part of the twentieth century, T2D was rare in people under age 20 and in pregnant women. In the United States, among Asian/Pacific Islanders and African-Americans, T2D is more prevalent than type 1 diabetes in adolescence. In 2000, 5.2% of deaths globally were due to T2D. In the United States, T2D is the leading cause of adult blindness, 60% of nontraumatic limb amputations, and 44% of end-stage renal failure [2].

5.3   Pathophysiology

Insulin resistance exists when the action of insulin is less than expected in terms of glucose uptake into cells and suppression of gluconeogenesis by the liver. Normally the pancreas is able to adapt to changes in insulin action as well as the amount of hyperglycemia. In T2D patients are unable to secrete enough insulin to overcome insulin resistance and to compensate for hyperglycemia.

β-cell dysfunction is believed to be one cause of insulin deficiency in T2D. The concepts of glucose toxicity and lipotoxicity to β-cells imply that irreversible damage to β-cells develops over time due to exposure to high levels of glucose or free fatty acids or both [3]. Progressive deterioration of insulin secretion is seen in most patients with T2D. Preservation of β-cell function is one of the goals of treatment.

5.4   Genetics/Heredity

T2D is considered a polygenic multifactorial disorder resulting from the interaction of multiple genes and environmental factors. If one parent has T2D, the lifetime risk to the offspring is 40%. That number is increased to 70% if both parents have T2D. In monozygotic twins, between 35 and 58% are concordant for T2D [3].

Linkage studies are studies of genes that are located near each other on the chromosome and tend to be inherited together. Linkage studies have identified two genes, CAPN10 and TCF7L2, which are associated with T2D.

TCF7L2 is on chromosome 10q. It was originally mapped in Mexican-Americans but has now been confirmed in other populations [2, 3].

CAPN10 is found on chromosome 2 in the NIDDM1 region. It encodes a cysteine protease. Single-nucleotide polymorphism of CAPN10 is associated with T2D and may also affect insulin sensitivity or secretion [3].

Genome-wide association studies have identified more than 40 genetic variants associated with T2D.

It is estimated that only 10% of T2D can be explained by the genes now known. Physical inactivity and excessive caloric intake are more sensitive predictors of T2D than genotype.

5.5   Diagnosis of T2D

- A1C ≥ 6.5% OR
- Fasting plasma glucose ≥126 mg/dL OR
- A 2 hour value ≥200 mg/dL after a 75 g oral glucose challenge OR
- A random plasma glucose ≥200 mg/dL in a patient with symptoms

High-risk women meeting the criteria cited above at the first prenatal visit can be given a diagnosis of overt diabetes diagnosed during pregnancy [4]. Testing for undiagnosed type 2 diabetes either before 13 weeks or at the first prenatal visit in high-risk patients is endorsed by the Endocrine Society and the ADA.

5.6   Prediabetes

Since 1997 the Expert Committee on the Diagnosis and Classification of Diabetes Mellitus has recognized a group of patients who have a level of glucose intolerance that does not meet the criteria for the diagnosis of T2D yet is too high to be considered normal. These patients are designated as having impaired fasting glucose (IFG) or impaired glucose tolerance (IGT) [4–6].
IFG = fasting 100–125 mg/dL
IGT = a 2 h value 140–199 mg/dL after a 75 g oral glucose load
A1C between 5.7 and 6.4%
The CDC estimates that one in three adult Americans has prediabetes. 15–30% will develop type 2 diabetes within 5 years.

5.7   Management in Pregnancy

Evaluation of end-organ status and a review of all medications should be conducted at the first prenatal visit. Evaluation of end-organ status should include a Hgb A1C to assess glycemic control over the last 3 months and during the period of organogenesis, an EKG to evaluate the heart, a 24 h urine collection to evaluate the amount of protein spillage and the creatinine clearance, an eye exam to rule out retinopathy if one has not been done within the last year, and a foot exam to rule out nonhealing wounds.

Review medications at the first visit to identify medications which should be discontinued and to identify patients who may need counseling regarding medications taken during the first trimester.

Accurate dating is critical in diabetes, and a dating sonogram should be ordered preferably in the first trimester. This should be followed by an anatomy sonogram including a complete fetal echocardiogram at 18–22 weeks to rule out congenital anomalies. Growth scans should be obtained monthly after 24 weeks.

The major goal of treatment of T2D is to prevent complications of the disease. During pregnancy, additional goals are to prevent fetal and neonatal morbidity and mortality. The best way to do this is by maintaining euglycemia. Dietary counseling and exercise are the first-line treatment followed by oral agents and insulin as a last resort.

Pregnant patients with T2D should check blood glucose four times each day, fasting and either one hour or two hours after each meal.

In nonpregnant patients, testing at this frequency is not required. Management of blood glucose is based on the hemoglobin A1c (HA1c). In nonpregnant patients, keeping the HA1c between 5 and 7% has been correlated with reduced development of retinopathy, neuropathy, and other complications of diabetes. These complications are not the primary concern during pregnancy. The primary concern is the fetus. HA1c has not been correlated with fetal outcomes. However, it must be noted that the level of glycemic control required in pregnancy is associated with a significant reduction in the risk for complications of diabetes. The benefit therefore is twofold.

Glycemic goals are fasting < 95 mg/dL and 1 h <140 mg/dL or 2 h <120 mg/dL.

When 20% of values for 2 consecutive weeks fail to meet goals, medication should be started. During pregnancy, oral agents may be used as the first-line treatment in appropriate patients with T2D. Glyburide may be considered, as well as metformin and acarbose. Oral agents will not achieve adequate control in patients with blood glucose much above 180mg/dL, and insulin will be required.

5.8   Prevention

Women with impaired glucose tolerance and/or gestational diabetes represent a group at high risk of progression to T2D. During pregnancy and postpartum are ideal times to identify this group of patients, provide education, and conduct necessary lifestyle interventions.

5.8.1   Breastfeeding

Breastfeeding lowers blood glucose and insulin concentration and may be associated with increased insulin sensitivity. There is noninsulin-mediated uptake of glucose to produce milk. Exclusive breastfeeding is associated with lower insulin levels and improved fasting glucose at 6–9 weeks postpartum. A longer duration of breastfeeding (>9 months) appears to lower the incidence of metabolic syndrome years after weaning. This effect was similar in all ethnic groups and for all ranges of BMI [7–9].

5.8.2   Lifestyle Modification

Lifestyle modification includes initiation of regular exercise, education, and dietary changes with the goal of sustainable weight loss. This has been shown to reduce the risk of T2D in women with a history of GDM by as much as 50% [10].

The CDC, as part of the National Diabetes Prevention Program, has created a lifestyle change program. This includes local programs that are approved by the CDC and an online program which is accessible to everyone. More details can be found at cdc.gov or by searching online for "lifestyle change program +CDC."

5.8.3   Medication

Several medications have been tested in an attempt to slow the progression from prediabetes or a history of GDM to T2D.

Metformin showed a 31% risk reduction in patients with prediabetes and a 50% risk reduction in patients with a history of GDM [11].

Acarbose showed a 25% reduction in risk in patients with IGT [12].

5.9 Summary

Type 2 diabetes is now considered a global health epidemic. Patients with type 2 diabetes are at increased risk of fetal anomalies, fetal macrosomia, neonatal hypoglycemia, and maternal preeclampsia. Goals of treatment are to prevent progression of the disease and to limit maternal and neonatal morbidity. Patients with prediabetes or a history of GDM are at risk of developing T2D. This group should be targeted for interventions to reduce progression to T2D.

References

1. Dunne F, Brydon P, Smith K, Gee H. Pregnancy in women with Type 2 diabetes: 12 years outcome data 1990–2002. Diabet Med. 2003;20(9):734–8.
2. Nolan CJ, Damm P, Prentki M. Type 2 diabetes across generations: from pathophysiology to prevention and management. Lancet. 2011;378(9786):169–81. doi:10.1016/S0140-6736(11)60614-4.
3. Stumvoll M, Goldstein BJ, van Haeften TW. Type 2 diabetes: principles of pathogenesis and therapy. Lancet. 2005;365(9467):1333–46. doi:10.1016/S0140-6736(05)61032-X.
4. American Diabetes Association. Diagnosis and classification of diabetes mellitus. Diabetes Care. 2010;33(Suppl 1):S62–9. doi:10.2337/dc10-S062.
5. The Expert Committee on the Diagnosis and Classification of Diabetes Mellitus. Report of the Expert Committee on the Diagnosis and Classification of Diabetes Mellitus. Diabetes Care. 1997;20(7):1183–97.
6. The Expert Committee on the Diagnosis and Classification of Diabetes Mellitus. Report of the Expert Committee on the

Diagnosis and Classification of Diabetes Mellitus. Diabetes Care. 2003;26(Suppl 1):S5–20.

7. Gunderson EP, Hedderson MM, Chiang V, Crites Y, Walton D, Azevedo RA, Fox G, Elmasian C, Young S, Salvador N, Lum M, Quesenberry CP, Lo JC, Sternfeld B, Ferrara A, Selby JV. Lactation intensity and postpartum maternal glucose tolerance and insulin resistance in women with recent GDM: the SWIFT cohort. Diabetes Care. 2012;35(1):50–6. doi:10.2337/dc11-1409.

8. Gunderson EP, Jacobs DR Jr, Chiang V, Lewis CE, Feng J, Quesenberry CP Jr, Sidney S. Duration of lactation and incidence of the metabolic syndrome in women of reproductive age according to gestational diabetes mellitus status: a 20-year prospective study in CARDIA (coronary artery risk development in young adults). Diabetes. 2010;59(2):495–504. doi:10.2337/db09-1197.

9. Stuebe AM, Kleinman K, Gillman MW, Rifas-Shiman SL, Gunderson EP, Rich-Edwards J. Duration of lactation and maternal metabolism at 3 years postpartum. J Women's Health. 2010;19(5):941–50. doi:10.1089/jwh.2009.1660.

10. Hod M, Hadar E, Cabero-Roura L. Prevention of type 2 diabetes among women with prior gestational diabetes mellitus. Int J Gynaecol Obstet. 2015;131(Suppl 1):S16–8. doi:10.1016/j.ijgo.2015.02.010.

11. Ratner RE, Christophi CA, Metzger BE, Dabelea D, Bennett PH, Pi-Sunyer X, Fowler S, Kahn SE, The Diabetes Prevention Program Research Group. Prevention of diabetes in women with a history of gestational diabetes: effects of metformin and lifestyle interventions. J Clin Endocrinol Metab. 2008;93(12):4774–9. doi:10.1210/jc.2008-0772.

12. Chiasson JL, Josse RG, Gomis R, Hanefeld M, Karasik A, Laakso M, Group S-NTR. Acarbose for prevention of type 2 diabetes mellitus: the STOP-NIDDM randomised trial. Lancet. 2002;359(9323):2072–7. doi:10.1016/S0140-6736(02)08905-5.

Chapter 6
Screening, Diagnosis, and Management of Gestational Diabetes

Lisa E. Moore

Fast Facts

- The best method of screening for gestational diabetes mellitus (GDM) is controversial.
- Diagnosis of type 2 diabetes during pregnancy is controversial.
- The American Diabetes Association (ADA), the International Association of Diabetes in Pregnancy Study Group (IADPSG), and the American College of Obstetricians and Gynecologist (ACOG) have each proposed different methods of diagnosis and screening.
- Depending on the method used, up to 25% of pregnancies in the United States are affected by GDM.

L.E. Moore, MD, FACOG
Department of Obstetrics and Gynecology, Texas Tech University
Health Sciences Center El Paso, Paul L. Foster School of Medicine,
El Paso, TX, USA
e-mail: lisa.e.moore@ttuhsc.edu

© Springer International Publishing AG 2018   45
L.E. Moore (ed.), *Diabetes in Pregnancy*,
https://doi.org/10.1007/978-3-319-65518-5_6

6.1   Introduction

Gestational diabetes mellitus (GDM) is glucose intolerance with onset or first recognition during pregnancy. This definition, though standard, is suitable only for categorization. During pregnancy, patients may have undiagnosed type 2 or, rarely, type 1 diabetes. They would still fall under the designation of GDM. This is problematic because the complications for both the mother and the fetus differ between GDM and preexisting diabetes. The definition does have the advantage of allowing a uniform approach to detection and classification of diabetes during pregnancy.

6.2   Why Should We Screen for GDM

The Hyperglycemia and Adverse Pregnancy Outcomes (HAPO) study was conducted at 15 centers in 9 countries. Data was collected and analyzed for 23,316 women who underwent a 75 g OGTT between 24 and 32 weeks. The study found a strong continuous association with maternal blood glucose levels lower than the level considered consistent with diabetes and poor maternal, fetal, and neonatal outcomes [1, 2].

Diabetes during the pregnancy increases the risk of preeclampsia, of macrosomia, and of neonatal hypoglycemia, hypocalcemia and respiratory distress [3, 4].

GDM increases the risk of type 2 diabetes. It has been projected that 50% of women with GDM will develop type 2 diabetes within 30 years of the index pregnancy. Hispanic women with a diagnosis of GDM have a 60% chance of developing type 2 diabetes within 5 years unless lifestyle modification is undertaken [4].

The concept of the "fetal origin of adult disease" or in utero programming indicates that the offspring of diabetic mothers are at increased risk of childhood obesity, metabolic syndrome, and type 2 diabetes [5, 6].

Identification of women with GDM represents an opportunity to disrupt the process of evolving glucose intolerance in the patient and in her children.

6.3 Screening/Diagnosis of GDM

The two-step screening process currently endorsed by ACOG was based on work by O'Sullivan and Mahan, who created cutoffs for diagnosing GDM based on a 100 g glucose load [7]. Interestingly these values were retrospectively validated based on their ability to predict future development of diabetes and were not related to fetal outcomes. In 1973 the same group introduced the 50 g load as a screening test and reported that a cutoff of 130 mg/dL was 79% sensitive and 87% specific for GDM. The values of the original O'Sullivan glucose tolerance test are still used today though they were modified in 1979 by the National Diabetes Data Group (NDDG) to adjust for the use of plasma instead of whole blood. Carpenter and Coustan used a more specific method of quantifying blood glucose and recommended using lower values as cutoffs [3].

Table 6.1 shows the original O'Sullivan values and the NDDG and Carpenter and Coustan values. Either NDDG or Carpenter and Coustan values can be used for the diagnosis of GDM. They are both endorsed by ACOG.

In 2010, the American Diabetes Association (ADA) working with the IADSP made the following recommendations for the diagnosis of GDM [8]:

- A fasting plasma glucose (FPG) > 126 mg/dL or a random blood glucose > 200 mg/dL is diagnostic of diabetes, and no glucose challenge is required.

TABLE 6.1 Diagnostic values after a 100 g OGTT

	O'Sullivan whole blood values	Values modified to use plasma (NDDG)	Carpenter and Coustan modification
Fasting		105	95
1 h	165	190	180
2 h	143	165	155
3 h	127	145	140

- Either one-step testing using the 75 g 2 h oral glucose tolerance test (OGTT) or the two-step approach currently used in the United States can be used to diagnose GDM.

In 2013, the World Health Organization (WHO) gave guidelines for the diagnosis of overt diabetes during pregnancy and for the diagnosis of GDM [9].

To diagnose overt diabetes in pregnancy, one or more of the following criteria must be met:

Fasting plasma glucose ≥ 126 mg/dL
Two hour plasma glucose ≥ 200 mg/dL after a 75 g glucose load
A random plasma glucose ≥ 200 mg/dL in the presence of symptoms of diabetes

WHO additionally recommended that GDM should be diagnosed at any time in pregnancy if one or more of the following criteria are met:

- Fasting plasma glucose of 92–125 mg/dL (note 126 mg/dL is indicative of preexisting diabetes)
- One hour plasma glucose ≥ 180 mg/dL after a 75 g load
- Two hour plasma glucose between 153 and 199 mg/dL after a 75 g glucose load

These values were adopted from the IADPSG consensus panel [10] and are endorsed by the American Diabetes Association (ADA). They were chosen based on the odds ratio of 1.75 for adverse neonatal events such as macrosomia, elevated C-peptide levels, and percent body fat >90th percentile.

Currently in the United States, the American College of Obstetricians and Gynecologists (ACOG) has not adopted one-step testing. It is worth pointing out that the lack of a worldwide consensus on the diagnosis of diabetes in pregnancy significantly limits the ability to define the worldwide prevalence of GDM and makes comparisons between studies that use different difficult criteria.

Conclusions of the 2013 NIH consensus on diagnosing gestation diabetes were that two-step testing identified

5–6% of the population as having GDM. The use of the 75 g 1 h test would increase the prevalence of GDM to 15–20%. It is not known whether these additional women would actually benefit from treatment. They concluded that there was not sufficient evidence to support adoption of the one-step testing [11].

In 2014 the United States Preventive Services Task Force (USPSTF) endorsed both two-step and one-step testing [12].

6.4 Who to Screen for GDM

Universal vs targeted screening.

Universal: every pregnant woman without known preexisting diabetes is screened.

Targeted: screen only those women with risk factors. Risk factors for GDM are shown in Table 6.2.

Due to the possible complications of undiagnosed gestational diabetes, universal screening is recommended.

TABLE 6.2 Risk factors for GDM

Two or more are considered high risk for GDM
Advanced maternal age
Obesity
Ethnicity (highest to lowest – Native American, Asian, Hispanic, African American, non-Hispanic White)
GDM in previous pregnancy
Previous macrosomic infant
Previous unexplained fetal death
Previous polyhydramnios
Polycystic ovarian syndrome
Metabolic syndrome
First degree relative with type 2 diabetes

6.5   When to Screen for GDM

Screening is traditionally done between 24 and 28 weeks. Insulin resistance increases during the second trimester due to placental hormones and other physiologic adaptations of pregnancy [13].

Patients with a previous history of GDM, a body mass index ≥ 30, and known impaired glucose tolerance or members of high-risk ethnic groups should be screened at the first prenatal visit [2, 4]. The test should be repeated at 24–28 weeks if initially negative.

For women who fail the 1 h but pass the 3 h at 28 weeks, an additional 11% will fail the 3 h if repeated in 4–6 weeks. A repeat 3 h test should be considered for ultrasound-proven fetal growth >85%.

6.6   How to Screen for GDM

Screening for GDM can be performed by either one-step testing or two-step testing. If you fall under the umbrella of ACOG, the current recommendation is for two-step testing. The ADA supports one-step testing and the USPSTF endorses both.

6.6.1   Two-Step Testing

Step 1. Screening for GDM: Step 1 identifies women who may have GDM and should be given the diagnostic 3 h test. Step 1 consists of a 50 g oral glucose load. The patient does not have to be fasting. Technically it should be done after 3–5 days of a high-carbohydrate diet. Suggested cutoffs range from 130 to 140 mg/dL. A cutoff of 130 mg/dL or 135 mg/dL identifies more patients and should be used in populations with a high rate of diabetes.

Patients who meet or exceed the cutoff for step 1 then go to step 2.

Step 2: Diagnosis of GDM: Step 2 consists of a 100 g oral glucose load. Blood sugar is checked prior to receiving the glucose and at 1, 2, and 3 hours after the glucose load. The patient must be fasting. Table 6.1 shows the NDDG and Carpenter and Coustan values. Two or more values that meet or exceed the cutoffs are diagnostic of GDM. Table 6.3 provides an overview of the different criteria for diagnosing GDM worldwide.

6.6.2   One-Step Testing

The patient should be fasting. The fasting blood glucose is measured, and a 75 g oral glucose load is given. Blood glucose is then checked at 1 and 2 h. One abnormal value makes the diagnosis of GDM. Recommended cutoffs are fasting $\geq$ 92 mg/dL, 1 h $\geq$ 180 mg/dL, and 2 h $\geq$ 153 mg/dL.

6.7   Management

Patients with gestational diabetes should check their blood glucose four times each day: fasting and either 1 or 2 h after each meal.

Glycemic goals are fasting <95 mg/dL, 2 h postprandial < 120 mg/dL, or 1 h postprandial < 140 mg/dL.

Failure to meet these glycemic goals with appropriate diet and exercise requires the addition of medication. If 20% of all values or 20% of the values for a specific testing period (i.e., fasting or postprandial breakfast, lunch, or dinner) are above the glycemic goals for a consecutive 2 weeks, medication should be started.

Example 1: A patient checks blood glucose four times a day, and over a 7 day period, three of her fastings are high. She returns in 1 week and two of her fastings are high. This meets the rule that 20% of her values during a specific testing period (i.e., fasting) are abnormal for 2 consecutive weeks.

Example 2: A patient checks blood glucose four times a day, and over a 7 day period, her abnormal values are 5/7 fasting abnormal, 3/7 breakfast abnormal, 3/7 lunch abnormal, and 1/7 dinner abnormal. Her food diary was reviewed, and she was counseled about carbohydrate intake and advised to have 30 min of exercise each day. She returns in 1 week. She has reduced her carbohydrates and is walking 15–30 min a day. Her abnormal values for the 7 day period are 3/7 fasting abnormal, 3/7 breakfast abnormal, 1/7 lunch abnormal, and 2/7 dinner abnormal. Greater than 20% of her values for 2 consecutive weeks have been abnormal, and she is a candidate for medication.

This may seem very quick, and there is a tendency to wait another week or two to see what happens. Consider that 2 weeks is equivalent to 5% of the baby's total in utero life. Four weeks is 10% of the baby's total in utero life. The longer that medication is delayed the greater the length of time that the baby is exposed to high blood glucose.

6.8   Is There a Difference in Checking Preprandial or Postprandial?

Many endocrinologists recommend preprandial testing for nonpregnant patients. This allows bolus insulin to correct for any elevated blood glucose prior to the meal and to compensate for the carbohydrates in the planned meal. However it does not tell if the amount of insulin was correct or whether there is continued postprandial hyperglycemia. After a meal, blood glucose peaks in approximately 1 h and returns to preprandial levels in 2–3 h. If blood glucose is tested postprandial, it doesn't matter what the preprandial level was because if the postprandial level meets goal, then the amount of insulin or other medications taken was correct. More importantly elevated postprandial blood glucose is associated with the development of fetal macrosomia [3].

6.9 Medication

When 20% of values fail to meet goals, medication should be started. Insulin is considered the gold standard for treatment of diabetes and has traditionally been the first-line agent for treatment of hyperglycemia in pregnancy not managed with diet and exercise. In actual practice oral agents are usually the first-line agent rather than insulin. The use of oral agents has been associated with enhanced compliance due to both ease of use, no need to measure insulin into a syringe, and patient comfort, no need to inject medication [14].

Once patients are on medication, either insulin or an oral agent, they should receive monthly growth scans, and antennal testing should be initiated at 32 weeks.

Delivery should be considered at 38 weeks for patients with suboptimal glucose control on medication.

6.10 Summary

Universal screening for GDM is recommended due to the epidemic of obesity and diabetes worldwide. GDM can be diagnosed using either the two-step method or the one-step method. The two-step method consists of an initial screen with a 50 g glucose load followed by a diagnostic 100 g 3 h test.

The one-step method is a 75 g oral glucose load with blood glucose measures at fasting and 1 and 2 hours after administration.

Once diagnosed, patients should check blood glucose four times each day. Medication should be initiated when diet and exercise fail to control hyperglycemia.

Table 6.3 Diagnostic criteria for GDM

Committee	Guidelines			Comments
ACOG [15]	Two step testing at 24–28 weeks			1 h cutoff of 130 mg/dl identifies more people but some will be normal
	Step 1: 50 g load test in 1 h			140 mg/dl identifies fewer people but they are more likely to have glucose intolerance
	Nonfasting			For the 3 h, Coustan values identify 50% more patients
	Cutoff (130–140)			
	Step 2: 100 g load			
	Test fasting 1,2,3 h limits are			
		Coustan	NDDG	
	Fasting	95	105	
	1 h	180	190	
	2 h	155	165	
	3 h	140	140	
	ADA			
	2 abnormals make the dx			

IADP SG 2010 [10]	1 step 75 g 2 h OGTT	Using IADP guidelines ~18% of US women will have dx of GDM
	Fasting < 92 mg/dl	IADPSG also supports a dx of overt diabetes for a fasting ≥126 mg/dl
	1 h < 180 mg/dl	
	2 h < 153 mg/dl	
	1 abnormal makes the dx	

(continued)

Table 6.3 (continued)

Committee	Guidelines	Comments
ADA 2016 [16]	Supports either one-step or two-step testing	ACOG recommends 130–135 mg/dl in high prevalence populations
	One-step testing	Either carpenter and Coustan values or the NDDG values can be used
	75 g-OGTT	
	$F \geq 92$ mg/dl	
	1 h ≥ 180 mg/dl	
	2 h ≥ 153 mg/dl	
	Two step testing	
	(1) 50 g glucose load	
	1 h ≥ 140 – Go to step 2	
	(2) 100 g OGTT	
	C/C NDDG	
	F ≥ 95 mg/dl 105 mg/dl	
	1 h ≥ 180 mg/dl 190 mg/dl	
	2 h ≥ 155 mg/dl 165 mg/dl	
	3 h ≥ 140 mg/dl 145 mg/dl	

NICE 2015	2-h 75 g OGTT	www.Nice.Org.uk/guidance/ng3
	In women with risk factors	To convert mmol/l to mg/dl multiply by 18
	If GDM in previous pregnancy	
	Offer test at first visit and repeat at 24–28 weeks if necessary	
	If fasting $\geq$ 5.6 mmol/l (100 mg/dl)	
	OR	
	2-h $\geq$ 7.8 mmol/l	
	140 mg/dl	
USPSTF 2014 [12]	Either 1-step or 2-step testing may be used	

ACOG American College of Obstetricians and Gynecologists, *IADP* International Association of Diabetes in Pregnancy, *ADA* American Diabetes Association, *NICE* National Institute for Health and Care Excellence (UK), *USPSTF* United States Preventive Service Task Force

References

1. Group HSCR, Metzger BE, Lowe LP, Dyer AR, Trimble ER, Chaovarindr U, Coustan DR, Hadden DR, McCance DR, Hod M, McIntyre HD, Oats JJ, Persson B, Rogers MS, Sacks DA. Hyperglycemia and adverse pregnancy outcomes. N Engl J Med. 2008;358(19):1991–2002. doi:10.1056/NEJMoa0707943.
2. McIntyre HD, Colagiuri S, Roglic G, Hod M. Diagnosis of GDM: a suggested consensus. Best Pract Res Clin Obstet Gynaecol. 2015;29(2):194–205. doi:10.1016/j.bpobgyn.2014.04.022.
3. Coustan DR. Gestational diabetes mellitus. Clin Chem. 2013;59(9):1310–21. doi:10.1373/clinchem.2013.203331.
4. Committee on Practice B-O. Practice Bulletin No. 137: gestational diabetes mellitus. Obstet Gynecol. 2013;122(2 Pt 1):406–16. doi:10.1097/01.AOG.0000433006.09219.f1.
5. Rizzo T, Metzger BE, Burns WJ, Burns K. Correlations between antepartum maternal metabolism and child intelligence. N Engl J Med. 1991;325(13):911–6. doi:10.1056/NEJM199109263251303.
6. Dabelea D, Mayer-Davis EJ, Lamichhane AP, D'Agostino RB Jr, Liese AD, Vehik KS, Narayan KM, Zeitler P, Hamman RF. Association of intrauterine exposure to maternal diabetes and obesity with type 2 diabetes in youth: the SEARCH case-control study. Diabetes Care. 2008;31(7):1422–6. doi:10.2337/dc07-2417.
7. O'Sullivan JB, Mahan CM. Criteria for the oral glucose tolerance test in pregnancy. Diabetes. 1964;13:278–85.
8. American Diabetes Association. Diagnosis and classification of diabetes mellitus. Diabetes Care. 2010;33(Suppl 1):S62–9. doi:10.2337/dc10-S062.
9. Diagnostic criteria and classification of hyperglycaemia first detected in pregnancy. Geneva 2013.
10. International Association of Diabetes, Pregnancy Study Groups Consensus Panel, Metzger BE, Gabbe SG, Persson B, Buchanan TA, Catalano PA, Damm P, Dyer AR, Leiva A, Hod M, Kitzmiler JL, Lowe LP, McIntyre HD, Oats JJ, Omori Y, Schmidt MI. International association of diabetes and pregnancy study groups recommendations on the diagnosis and classification of hyperglycemia in pregnancy. Diabetes Care. 2010;33(3):676–82. doi:10.2337/dc09-1848.
11. Vandorsten JP, Dodson WC, Espeland MA, Grobman WA, Guise JM, Mercer BM, Minkoff HL, Poindexter B, Prosser LA, Sawaya

GF, Scott JR, Silver RM, Smith L, Thomas A, Tita AT. NIH consensus development conference: diagnosing gestational diabetes mellitus. NIH Consens State Sci Statements. 2013;29(1):1–31.

12. Moyer VA, Force USPST. Screening for gestational diabetes mellitus: U.S. preventive services task force recommendation statement. Ann Intern Med. 2014;160(6):414–20. doi:10.7326/M13-2905.

13. Rani PR, Begum J. Screening and diagnosis of gestational diabetes mellitus, where do we stand. J Clin Diagn Res. 2016;10(4):QE01–4. doi:10.7860/JCDR/2016/17588.7689.

14. Rowan JA, Hague WM, Gao W, Battin MR, Moore MP, Mi GTI. Metformin versus insulin for the treatment of gestational diabetes. N Engl J Med. 2008;358(19):2003–15. doi:10.1056/NEJMoa0707193.

15. Committee Opinion No. 504. Screening and diagnosis of gestational diabetes mellitus. Obstet Gynecol. 2011;118(3):751–3. doi:10.1097/AOG.0b013e3182310cc3.

16. American Diabetes Association. Standards of medical Care in Diabetes-2016 abridged for primary care providers. Clin Diabetes. 2016;34(1):3–21. doi:10.2337/diaclin.34.1.3.

Chapter 7
Prenatal Care for the Pregnant Diabetic Patient

Lisa E. Moore

Fast Facts

- All patients should check blood glucose a minimum of four times a day: fasting and after each meal.
- Glycemic goals are fasting ≤95 mg/dL and 2 h postprandial ≤120 mg/dL and 1 h postprandial ≤140 mg/dL.
- Patients with diabetes are at increased risk of developing preeclampsia.

7.1 Introduction

The ultimate goal of all prenatal care is a healthy baby and a healthy mother. Prenatal care achieves this goal by modifying known risk factors for adverse outcomes when possible such as treating hyperglycemia and by identifying developing

L.E. Moore, MD, FACOG
Department of Obstetrics and Gynecology, Texas Tech University
Health Sciences Center El Paso, Paul L. Foster School of Medicine,
El Paso, TX, USA
e-mail: lisa.e.moore@ttuhsc.edu

© Springer International Publishing AG 2018   61
L.E. Moore (ed.), *Diabetes in Pregnancy*,
https://doi.org/10.1007/978-3-319-65518-5_7

events that require intervention (e.g., preeclampsia). For patients with diabetes, the goals of prenatal care are to maintain normoglycemia to prevent the development of macrosomia and to avoid neonatal complications such as respiratory distress, hypoglycemia, and shoulder dystocia.

7.2   Daily Self-Monitoring of Blood Glucose

All patients should be given a prescription for a glucometer, lancets, and test strips.

Test strips are specific to the glucometer.

There are several software programs which can be used to download the recorded blood glucose levels from the glucometer. Those programs are usually meter specific or manufacturer specific, so some sites prefer that all the patients in their clinics use the same type of glucometer. Most manufacturers offer free software on their website. There are also proprietary products for purchase that work with multiple makes of glucometers and allow creation of a database of patients.

At initial diagnosis, patients should be referred for dietary counseling and teaching on how to use the glucometer to test blood glucose levels.

For gestational diabetics and type 2 diabetics, it is recommended to test four (4) times a day: fasting and after breakfast, after lunch, and after dinner. Postprandial levels of hyperglycemia have been shown to more closely correlate with the development of macrosomia. There is controversy around whether it is best to test at 1 h postprandial or at 2 h. A randomized trial in which 66 women were assigned to check at 1 h postprandial and 46 women were assigned to check at 2 h postprandial found that checking at 1 h was associated with decreased requirement for insulin therapy but no difference in neonatal or obstetric outcomes [1].

One hour postprandial blood glucose should be 140 mg/dL or less. Two hour postprandial blood glucose should be 120 mg/dL or less. Fasting should be 95 mg/dL or less.

Patients with type 1 diabetes should check fasting blood glucose and preprandial and postprandial blood glucose (i.e., seven times daily at a minimum). The preprandial glucose is used to correct for any hyperglycemia present before the meal. Preprandial blood glucose should be 60–100 mg/dL. Type 1 diabetics will inject insulin prior to eating that will correct for the carbohydrates they are about to eat and the degree of hyperglycemia noted in the preprandial check. The postprandial check confirms the accuracy of the preprandial insulin dose and allows correction if needed.

Continuous glucose monitoring has been studied in pregnant women with preexisting diabetes. There are several continuous monitors on the market, and this may be the way that diabetes will be monitored in the future. The literature is evolving on the ways that continuous monitoring may improve outcomes.

7.3   Ultrasound Evaluation

Patients with gestational diabetes managed with diet and exercise alone should have an ultrasound at 18–22 weeks to evaluate anatomy. No additional ultrasounds are recommended unless there are concerns about fetal growth.

Patients with gestational diabetes requiring medication, type 2 diabetes, or type 1 diabetes should have an anatomy ultrasound at 18–22 weeks and an evaluation of fetal growth on a monthly basis thereafter.

Accurate pregnancy dating is particularly important in diabetic patients due the risk of growth abnormalities. Ideally a dating scan should be obtained in the first trimester. However a scan up to 20 weeks is considered accurate dating.

The evaluation of fetal anatomy is particularly important in patients with preexisting diabetes to rule out congenital anomalies. It should be performed as close to 20 weeks as possible and should include an expert evaluation of the fetal heart to rule out the presence of a cardiac anomaly.

7.4   Antenatal Testing

Antenatal testing can be performed in a variety of ways:

- Nonstress test (NST)—two episodes of an increase in amplitude of the heart rate by 15 beats per minute, lasting for 15 seconds, in 20 min are considered reactive.
- Modified biophysical profile (BPP) consists of an NST and evaluation of the amniotic fluid index (AFI).
- Biophysical profile includes an NST, three episodes of gross body movement, breathing for 30 s, one episode of flexion and extension, and a 2 cm × 2 cm pocket of amniotic fluid. Each item is scored either 0(absent) or 2(present). The maximum score is 10.

The NST is equivalent to the BPP in sensitivity to fetal acidosis. The NST is the first parameter to demonstrate change when the fetus is becoming acidotic. Addition of an AFI to the NST (i.e., the modified BPP) is less time-consuming to perform and allows assessment of an acute indicator (the NST) and a chronic indicator (fluid) of the fetal well-being.

Type 1 diabetes initiate testing at 28 weeks.
Type 2 diabetes initiate testing 28–32 weeks. Start at 28 weeks if glycemic control is poor.

Gestational diabetes:

A1 GDM who by default have good glycemic control—no recommendation.
A2 GDM initiate testing at 28–32 weeks. Start at 28 weeks if control is poor.

7.5   Laboratory Evaluation

Patients with preexisting diabetes should be evaluated for end-organ damage.

A1C—provides an indication of the degree of glycemic control over the last 3 months.

An A1C of 8%, indicating that 8% of RBCs are glycosylated, is associated with an average blood glucose of 180 mg/dL.

For each 1% above or below 8, add or subtract 30 mg/dL to estimate the associated average blood glucose level.

Twenty-four hour urine collection to determine if and how much protein is being spilled and the creatinine clearance. Protein spillage is indicator of damage to the kidneys and will provide a baseline for future evaluation for preeclampsia. Creatinine clearance should be 150 mL/s or greater during pregnancy.

Eye exam to rule out retinopathy.

EKG to detect rhythm abnormalities may also detect heart enlargement, axis deviation, or subtle changes in function.

Foot examination—particularly in type 1 diabetics and in poorly controlled type 2 diabetics. Foot injuries due to relatively poor circulation and a hyperglycemic environment may be slow to heal and can lead to damage or amputations. Pay special attention to ingrown toenails. They can lead to amputation in patients with diabetes.

Dentist—patients should be asked if they have dental concerns and referred to a dentist as indicated. Dental abscesses can cause loss of glucose control in type 1 and type 2 patients both because of inability to eat and because of the infection. Dental abscesses can precipitate DKA in type 1 diabetic patients.

Routine prenatal labs (should be done at the first prenatal visit):

Type and screen
Hemoglobin-hematocrit
Gonorrhea screening
Chlamydia screening
HIV screening
RPR
Hepatitis B
Review pap smear

7.6   Serum Screening for Aneuploidy

Cell-free DNA should be offered to high-risk women and can be done as early as 10 weeks.

At the time of this writing, ACOG has not approved its use in low-risk women; however, the American College of

Medical Genetics and Genomics recommends both low-risk and high-risk women should be offered the test [2, 3]. If cell-free DNA testing is performed, it does not screen for neural tube defects. The maternal serum alpha-feto-protein (MSAFP) must be ordered at the standard 16–20 weeks.

Maternal serum screening at 16–20 weeks should be performed to provide a risk assessment for aneuploidy and to screen for neural tube defects. It is not necessary to do both cell-Free DNA and serum screening.

7.7   Delivery

A1 GDM, by definition, are well controlled and can be allowed to labor spontaneously. If induction of labor is considered, it should be after 39 weeks.

A2 GDM with good control may also be allowed to labor spontaneously or may be induced after 39 weeks. Patients with poor control should be induced at 38 weeks.

Type 2 and type 1 diabetics should plan delivery at 38 weeks.

7.8   Postpartum

GDM A1 and A2

> 75 g 2 h glucose tolerance test
> Performed while fasting
> 2 h value ≤ 139 mg/dL normal

> 140–199 mg/dL impaired glucose tolerance
> ≥200 mg/dL consistent with diabetes

> Type 1 and Type 2

> Follow up with primary care provider for management of diabetes.

	A1 GDM	A2 GDM	Preexisting diabetes
First visit	Routine labs	Routine labs	• Routine labs
			• 24 h urine
			• Eye exam to r/o retinopathy
			• EKG
			• Ask about dentist and foot injuries
10 weeks	Cell-free DNA screen	Cell-free DNA screen	Cell-free DNA screen
16–20 weeks	Serum marker screen	Serum marker screen	Serum marker screen
18–22 weeks	Anatomy scan	Anatomy scan	Anatomy scan and fetal echo
26–32 weeks	Growth scan	Initiate monthly growth scan	Initiate monthly growth scan
32 weeks	Routine	Weekly NST/AFI	Weekly NST/AFI
Delivery	May labor spontaneously	If good control deliver by 40 weeks. If poor control deliver at 38 weeks	Deliver at 38 weeks

References

1. Weisz B, Shrim A, Homko CJ, Schiff E, Epstein GS, Sivan E. One hour versus two hours postprandial glucose measurement in gestational diabetes: a prospective study. J Perinatol: official

journal of the California Perinatal Association. 2005;25(4):241–4. doi:10.1038/sj.jp.7211243.

2. Committee Opinion Summary No. 640. Cell-free DNA screening for fetal aneuploidy. Obstet Gynecol. 2015;126(3):691–2. doi:10.1097/01.AOG.0000471171.86798.ac.

3. Gregg AR, Skotko BG, Benkendorf JL, Monaghan KG, Bajaj K, Best RG, Klugman S, Watson MS. Noninvasive prenatal screening for fetal aneuploidy, 2016 update: a position statement of the American College of Medical Genetics and Genomics. Genet Med. 2016;18(10):1056–65. doi:10.1038/gim.2016.97.

Chapter 8
Patient Education

Diana Clokey and Lisa E. Moore

> **Fast Facts**
>
> - Addressing the psychological adjustment to the diagnosis of diabetes is an essential part of diabetes education.
> - Family members should be included in diabetes education.

8.1 Introduction

Patient education is an essential component in the treatment of diabetes. An informed and motivated patient contributes to improved outcomes. Unless the patient understands the disease, the possible consequences, and the methods to

D. Clokey, MSRD, RPH, CDE (✉)
Albuquerque, NM, USA
e-mail: clokeydiana@gmail.com

L.E. Moore, MD, FACOG
Department of Obstetrics and Gynecology, Texas Tech University Health Sciences Center El Paso, Paul L. Foster School of Medicine, El Paso, TX, USA
e-mail: lisa.e.moore@ttuhsc.edu

© Springer International Publishing AG 2018   69
L.E. Moore (ed.), *Diabetes in Pregnancy*,
https://doi.org/10.1007/978-3-319-65518-5_8

control the disease and reduce the risk of complications, management is likely to be unsuccessful. It is true that an informed patient may choose to disregard appropriate diabetes-related behaviors, but an uneducated patient fails through lack of knowledge rather than by choice. A team approach to care is recognized as optimal. In addition to the patient, other essential team members are the physician, the certified diabetic educator, and the registered dietician.

Typically, patients with a new diagnosis of diabetes during pregnancy attend a group class in which they are provided general information on diabetes, a discussion of the psychological adjustment to the diagnosis of diabetes, instructions on carbohydrate counting and label reading, dietary guidelines, and appropriate exercise, and they are taught how to program the glucometer and how to test blood glucose. Patients who subsequently require medication to achieve euglycemia are taught about the medications and instructed on insulin use as needed at clinic appointments or in a classroom setting.

8.2   General Information on Diabetes

- General definition of diabetes mellitus [1]:
- Type 1 diabetes is due to insufficient endogenous production of insulin.
- Type 2 diabetes is insulin resistance-mediated glucose intolerance.
- Gestational diabetes is glucose intolerance first recognized during pregnancy, mediated by insulin resistance, and may lead to type 2 diabetes.
- Possible risks and complications to the mother[2]:

  - Increased risk of preeclampsia
  - Increased risk of cesarean delivery

- Possible risks to the baby [3–5]:

  - Congenital anomalies in pre-existing diabetes with poor control
  - Macrosomia

- – Birth injury
- – Stillbirth
- – Neonatal jaundice
- – Programming for obesity and early onset type 2 diabetes

- Chronic complications that can develop from poorly controlled diabetes [6–10]:

  - – Retinopathy
  - – Amputations
  - – Peripheral neuropathy
  - – Renal dysfunction
  - – Cardiovascular disease
  - – Increased risk of Alzheimer's

- Importance of receiving ongoing medical care during pregnancy, 6-week postpartum visit, and follow-up care with primary physician after delivery

8.3   Psychological Adjustment

- A diagnosis of diabetes can be a significant life stressor. The necessary lifestyle changes impact not just the patient but her family and acquaintances. There can be stress at work if the patient is not allowed to eat when needed or to check blood glucose. Patients with chaotic lives—those who are homeless or working more than one job—or with limited resources, who don't typically maintain a schedule, will find it difficult to adhere to diet and testing regimens.
- Family members need to be included to provide support and encouragement to the patient. Patients often relate that they have to cook one meal for the family and something different for themselves to maintain the diet. This can also be a financial stressor if it is necessary to buy different food. Educating the family members on the importance of the diet will enhance compliance.
- Social workers and nurse case manager can provide support through counseling and addressing socioeconomic issues.
- In certain circumstances a referral to a psychologist may be appropriate.

8.4 Nutrition

- Nutrition is arguably the most important component of patient education.
- Patients should be instructed on carbohydrate counting and label reading:

    - One serving of carbohydrate is 15 g. Three to four carbohydrate servings per meal are recommended.

- Patients should keep a food diary which is reviewed at each visit.
- Discuss appropriate weight gain for pregnancy based on Institute of medicine recommendations. Women who are morbidly obese, BMI ≥35, may improve birth outcome by gaining little or no weight during pregnancy [11].
- An Individual meal plan should be developed, with the help of a dietician, to provide adequate calories and nutrients to support a healthy pregnancy.

8.5 Exercise

- Women who are physically active before and in early pregnancy have a lower rate of gestational diabetes.
- In absence of either medical or obstetric complications, 30 min or more of moderate exercise a day on most, if not all, days of the week is recommended for pregnant women [12].
- Safe forms of exercises include walking, swimming, water aerobics, yoga for pregnancy, and upper extremity exercise when patient is assigned bed rest.
- Women with pre-existing diabetes should monitor their blood glucose before, during, and after exercise. A small snack prior to exercise may be appropriate.

8.6 Medication

- Oral agents

    - Instruction on type, dose, and potential side effects of medication

- Insulin

  - Instruction on injection technique and rotation of sites, knowledge of which insulins may be mixed and how to mix them

- How to read the markings on an insulin syringe and how to draw up insulin

  - Insulin syringes: 1/3 cc (30 units) with half-unit increments, 1/2 cc (50 units) with one-unit increments, and 1 cc syringe (100 units) with two-unit increments

- Storage and care of insulin. Correct disposal of needles

  - Unopened insulin should be refrigerated. Opened insulin can be kept at room temperature for 28 days. High temperatures will decrease efficacy.

- Alternative insulin delivery systems such as insulin pens, needle-less injectors, and insulin pumps

8.7   Monitoring Blood Glucose Levels

- Daily self-monitoring of blood glucose is necessary to achieve euglycemia.
- Glycemic goals should be set, and the patient should know what the goals are [2]:

  - Fasting $\leq$95 mg/dl
  - One hour postprandial $\leq$140 mg/dl
  - Two hour postprandial $\leq$120 mg/dl

- Patients should be aware of when to test blood glucose:

  - GDM and type 2 check should test four times a day, at fasting and 1 or 2 h.
  - Postprandial.
  - Type 1 DM test fasting, pre- and post-meal, plus HS and 3 am when necessary.
  - Additional testing during exercise and on sick days should be discussed.

- Instruction on how to test blood glucose:
  - Wash hands with soap and water prior to testing.
  - Test on sides of fingers not the tips.
  - Rotate testing sites.
  - Limit use of alcohol swabs because they can dry the skin and cause cracking.
  - Some hand lotions may cause a falsely elevated reading.
- Proper disposal of lancets and test strips:
  - A small "sharps container" may be purchased at a pharmacy, or the patient may use a metal or heavy plastic container that can be properly sealed before disposal.

8.8   Acute Complications

8.8.1   Hypoglycemia

- The patient and family members should understand the causes of hypoglycemia:
  - Taking too much insulin
  - Taking medication and not eating
  - Exercise
- The patient and family members should know the symptoms of hypoglycemia:

Sweating	Thirst
Nausea and vomiting	Tingling in lips and mouth
Shakiness or tremor	Headache
Anxiety	Extreme hunger
Heart palpitations	Loss of consciousness
Confusion	Seizures

- The patient and family members should understand the treatment for hypoglycemia:
  - In an emergency give any sugar on hand (juice, candy, soft drinks).
  - Do not give liquid or food to an unconscious person.

- With mild symptoms can use glucose tablets or saltine crackers and milk:

  - For mild symptoms the goal is to alleviate symptoms without overshooting into hyperglycemia.
  - It takes about 15 min to see the effect of glucose given to correct hypoglycemia.
  - Rule of 15: Take 15 grams of carbohydrate every 15 min until blood glucose reaches 100.
  - Examples of 15 g of carbohydrate: half cup orange juice, five to six Life Savers candies, 8 oz. glass of milk, four glucose tablets, and four to six saltine crackers.

- Hypoglycemia unawareness is a severe complication of diabetes in which patients do not experience the typical symptoms of hypoglycemia and will fail to take corrective action. This may result in seizures, loss of consciousness, and death. It is more common in patients who have chronic poor control.

8.9   Hyperglycemia

- The patient and family members should understand the causes of hyperglycemia:

  - Illness
  - Not taking medication (insulin or oral agents)
  - Incorrect dosing of medication
  - Noncompliance with diet

- The patient and family members should know the symptoms of hyperglycemia:

  - Frequent urination
  - Thirst
  - Fatigue/lethargy
  - Headache
  - Fruity odor on breath
  - Nausea and vomiting
  - Dyspnea
  - Confusion

- The patient and family members should understand how to treat hyperglycemia:

  - Mild hyperglycemia (<170) do nothing—walking may help.
  - Moderate hyperglycemia (170–250)—if on insulin, give a corrective dose using the correction factor.
  - Severe hyperglycemia (> 250)—give corrective insulin, if signs of DKA are present go to the hospital.

8.10   Sick Days

- During illness, maintenance of glycemic control will require adjustments in the frequency of self-blood glucose monitoring. Medication adjustments may also be required.
- Inform the patient who to contact for illness during which glycemic control is compromised.
- When patient is unable to eat usual diet because of illness:

  - For blood glucose ≥250 mg/dl: water, broth, diet drinks, ice chips, sugar-free gelatin, and sugar-free ice pops. Check in with provider and be alert for DKA.
  - For blood glucose <70 mg/dl: fruit juice, *not diet* ginger ale, 7-up and cola drinks, glucose tablets, ice pops, gelatin, soups, milk ice cream, and puddings.

8.11   Hygiene

- Instruction includes the importance of hygiene, skin care, and dental care.

8.12   Foot Care

- The risk for lower extremity amputation is high for persons with pre-existing diabetes:

  - Frequent foot exams (both self-examination and by the physician).
  - Appropriate foot care, including avoiding ingrown toenails, bunions, blisters, and sores that may have difficulty healing.

 – Appropriate shoe choices.
 – Referral to a podiatrist is recommended for baseline evaluation.
 – Regular follow-up.

8.13   Breastfeeding

• Breastfeeding is beneficial to both mother and baby.
• Benefits to the mother include [13–16]:

 – Weight loss:
 – Helps reduce or delay subsequent diabetes in women with GDM.
 – One year of breastfeeding decreased the rate of diabetes by 15% in the normal population of women.

• Benefits for offspring include [17–19]:

 – Decreased risk of sudden infant death syndrome (SIDS).
 – Fewer urinary tract and upper respiratory infections.
 – Lowers the lifetime risk of diabetes and obesity.

• Refer the patient to lactation resources as needed. A lactation clinic is commonly found in breastfeeding friendly hospitals.

8.14   Community Resources

• Patient should be made aware of resources that are available in the community for both pregnancy and diabetes.
• Resources for pregnancy such as Women, Infant, and Children (WIC) food supplement program, SAFE ride, and lactation clinic.
• After delivery, resources for women with GDM or pre-existing DM may be available through a hospital's patient education program, i.e., pre-diabetes class for GDM and DM classes for those diagnosed with pre-existing DM.
• Other groups include the American Diabetes Association and the Juvenile Diabetes foundation.

8.15 Postpartum

- Keeping the 6-week postpartum visit is important. Only about 50% of women keep their postpartum visit.
- Patients with GDM should receive 75 g GTT at the 6-week postpartum visit.[20]
- If the patient has an abnormal GTT, the appropriate referral should be made for follow-up for the patient's diabetes.
- The American Diabetes Association recommends a 1-year follow-up for blood glucose evaluation and then every 3 years for women who have had GDM.
- Women with pre-existing diabetes should return to the care of their primary provider.

8.16 Summary

Patient education about diabetes and diabetes management is one of the most important aspects of the care of the diabetic patient.

References

1. American Diabetes Association. Diagnosis and classification of diabetes mellitus. Diabetes Care. 2010;33(Suppl 1):S62–9. doi:10.2337/dc10-S062.
2. Benhalima K, Devlieger R, Van Assche A. Screening and management of gestational diabetes. Best Pract Res Clin Obstet Gynaecol. 2015;29(3):339–49. doi:10.1016/j.bpobgyn.2014.07.026.
3. Anderson JL, Waller DK, Canfield MA, Shaw GM, Watkins ML, Werler MM. Maternal obesity, gestational diabetes, and central nervous system birth defects. Epidemiology. 2005;16(1):87–92.
4. Hillier TA, Pedula KL, Schmidt MM, Mullen JA, Charles MA, Pettitt DJ. Childhood obesity and metabolic imprinting: the ongoing effects of maternal hyperglycemia. Diabetes Care. 2007;30(9):2287–92. doi:10.2337/dc06-2361.
5. Dabelea D, Mayer-Davis EJ, Lamichhane AP, D'Agostino RB Jr, Liese AD, Vehik KS, Narayan KM, Zeitler P, Hamman RF. Association of intrauterine exposure to maternal diabetes

and obesity with type 2 diabetes in youth: the SEARCH case-control study. Diabetes Care. 2008;31(7):1422–6. doi:10.2337/dc07-2417.

6. American Diabetes Association. Professional practice committee for the standards of medical care in diabetes-2016. Diabetes Care. 2016;39(Suppl 1):S107–8. doi:10.2337/dc16-S018.

7. Atkinson MA, Eisenbarth GS, Michels AW. Type 1 diabetes. Lancet. 2014;383(9911):69–82. doi:10.1016/S0140-6736(13)60591-7.

8. Bulletins ACoP. ACOG practice bulletin. Clinical management guidelines for obstetrician-gynecologists. Number 60, march 2005. Pregestational diabetes mellitus. Obstet Gynecol. 2005;105(3):675–85.

9. Dunne F, Brydon P, Smith K, Gee H. Pregnancy in women with type 2 diabetes: 12 years outcome data 1990-2002. Diabet Med. 2003;20(9):734–8.

10. Sutherland GT, Lim J, Srikanth V, Bruce DG. Epidemiological approaches to understanding the link between type 2 diabetes and dementia. J Alzheimers Dis. 2017;59(2):393–403. doi:10.3233/JAD-161194.

11. American College of Obstetricians and Gynecologists. ACOG Committee opinion no. 548: weight gain during pregnancy. Obstet Gynecol. 2013;121(1):210–2. doi:10.1097/01. AOG.0000425668.87506.4c.

12. ACOG Committee Opinion No. 650. Physical activity and exercise during pregnancy and the postpartum period. Obstet Gynecol. 2015;126(6):e135–42. doi:10.1097/AOG.0000000000001214.

13. Gunderson EP, Jacobs DR Jr, Chiang V, Lewis CE, Feng J, Quesenberry CP Jr, Sidney S. Duration of lactation and incidence of the metabolic syndrome in women of reproductive age according to gestational diabetes mellitus status: a 20-year prospective study in CARDIA (coronary artery risk development in young adults). Diabetes. 2010;59(2):495–504. doi:10.2337/db09-1197.

14. Stuebe AM, Kleinman K, Gillman MW, Rifas-Shiman SL, Gunderson EP, Rich-Edwards J. Duration of lactation and maternal metabolism at 3 years postpartum. J Women's Health. 2010;19(5):941–50. doi:10.1089/jwh.2009.1660.

15. Gunderson EP, Hedderson MM, Chiang V, Crites Y, Walton D, Azevedo RA, Fox G, Elmasian C, Young S, Salvador N, Lum M, Quesenberry CP, Lo JC, Sternfeld B, Ferrara A, Selby JV. Lactation intensity and postpartum maternal glucose tolerance and insulin resistance in women with recent GDM: the SWIFT cohort. Diabetes Care. 2012;35(1):50–6. doi:10.2337/dc11-1409.

16. Fox M, Berzuini C, Knapp LA. Maternal breastfeeding history and Alzheimer's disease risk. J Alzheimers Dis. 2013;37(4):809–21. doi:10.3233/JAD-130152.

17. Halipchuk J, Temple B, Dart A, Martin D, Sellers EAC. Prenatal, obstetric and perinatal factors associated with the development of childhood-onset type 2 diabetes. Can J Diabetes. 2017. doi: 10.1016/j.jcjd.2017.04.003

18. Bowatte G, Tham R, Allen KJ, Tan DJ, Lau M, Dai X, Lodge CJ. Breastfeeding and childhood acute otitis media: a systematic review and meta-analysis. Acta Paediatr. 2015;104(467):85–95. doi:10.1111/apa.13151.

19. Carlin RF, Moon RY. Risk factors, protective factors, and current recommendations to reduce sudden infant death syndrome: a review. JAMA Pediatr. 2017;171(2):175–80. doi:10.1001/jamapediatrics.2016.3345.

20. Committee on Practice Bulletins—Obstetrics. Practice bulletin no. 137: gestational diabetes mellitus. Obstet Gynecol. 2013;122(2 Pt 1):406–16. doi:10.1097/01.AOG.0000433006.09219.f1.

Chapter 9
The Diabetic Diet

Diana Clokey

Fast Facts

- One serving of carbohydrate is 15 g.
- Carbohydrate counting (reading labels) is essential for management of diabetes.

9.1 Introduction

The diabetic diet provides a way of eating to help control blood glucose and to maintain a healthy weight. During pregnancy the goal is to provide enough nutrients to support the developing baby while limiting episodes of hyperglycemia and avoiding the production of ketones. Surprisingly, specific dietary recommendations are poorly studied during pregnancy, and no data exists to support one dietary approach over another [1].

D. Clokey, MSRD, RPH, CDE
Albuquerque, NM, USA
e-mail: clokeydiana@gmail.com

© Springer International Publishing AG 2018
L.E. Moore (ed.), *Diabetes in Pregnancy*,
https://doi.org/10.1007/978-3-319-65518-5_9

9.2   General Nutrition Guidelines

- Avoid sugar, concentrated sweets, and refined/processed starches.
- Eliminate liquid carbohydrate (soda pop, energy drinks, juices) and test milk.
- Identify carbohydrate foods/label reading.
- Eat three meals plus three snacks.
- Emphasize higher protein and less carbohydrate at breakfast (cereal after 11 am).
- Encourage high-fiber foods.
- Limit high fat foods. Limit fast foods.
- Sugar substitutes. Safe when consumed with acceptable daily intakes established by the FDA [2].
- Encourage physical activity. 150 min per week of moderate intensity aerobic exercise is recommended [3].
- Monitor weight for appropriate weight gain.
- Refer to registered dietitian for medical nutritional therapy (MNT) and lifestyle changes.

9.3   Medical Nutrition Therapy (MNT)

MNT is the cornerstone of treatment. It is the only therapy for 40–58% of women with GDM.

- Distribution of macronutrients, 33–40% CHO, 20% PRO, and 40% FAT of total daily calories [3].
- Calorie requirements are based on height, prepregnancy weight, and level of activity.
- Most pregnant women require 2200–2900 Kcal per day.
- Recommend increase in calories per trimester is [4]:

First trimester	0
Second trimester	340 kcal
Third trimester	452 kcal

- Recommendations for women with multiple gestations are extrapolated from singleton gestations. An additional 300 calories per day per additional fetus is recommended [5].

9.4   Carbohydrate

- Minimum amount of carbohydrate per day required in pregnancy is 175 grams. Amount of carbohydrate typically found in an 1800 calorie diet [4].
- Main energy source for the body. One hundred percent of carbohydrate is converted into glucose during digestion.
- Simple carbohydrates are absorbed quickly and should be avoided except when treating a hypoglycemic reaction.
- Simple carbohydrates include, for example, table sugar, candy, syrup, jelly, honey, regular soft drinks, energy drinks, Gatorade, and fruit juice. In limited amounts milk and fruit are allowed.
- Complex carbohydrates (starch and fiber) breakdown slower compared to simple carbohydrates and are allowed in measured amounts [6, 7].
- Complex carbohydrates include, for example, whole grain/multi-grain products (bread, tortillas, rice, crackers, pasta, cereals) and starchy vegetables (pinto beans/legumes, potatoes, corn, peas, and sweet potatoes). Avoid white refined flours and instant cereals and noodles. Limit processed foods and fast foods. Unsweetened cereals to be eaten after 11 am.

9.5   Protein and Fat

- Both protein and fat contain no carbohydrate and take longer to breakdown in the body. Approximately 58% of protein and 10% of fat are converted to glucose during digestion.
- Foods in both these categories, plus the non-starchy vegetables, help provide adequate calories and nutrients for the pregnancy.
- Protein food sources include meat, poultry, fish, cheese, cottage cheese, nuts, nut butters, and tofu.
- Fat food sources include oil, butter, margarine, mayonnaise, cream, sour cream, and avocados. Encourage more mono-/polyunsaturated fat instead of saturated fat.

- Low-carbohydrate vegetables include lettuce, tomatoes, cucumber, peppers, carrots, broccoli, green beans, chili, asparagus, etc.

9.6   Carbohydrate Budget

Carbohydrate is the primary macronutrient that has the greatest impact on glucose levels. Therefore, the amount of carbohydrate is distributed throughout the day into three meals and three snacks. A serving of carbohydrate = 15 grams of carbohydrate. This is the amount of carbohydrate in an 8 oz. glass of milk, a slice of bread, half cup of noodles, or a small piece of fresh fruit. Table 9.1 shows how carbohydrate intake should be distributed over a typical day.

TABLE 9.1 Daily carbohydrate budget with examples

Time	CHO servings	Grams of CHO	Example
Breakfast	1–2 servings	15–30 g	Two pieces of toast, margarine, eggs, bacon, hot tea (decaf)
Midmorning snack	1–2 servings	15–30 g	Four to six crackers, cheese, small fresh fruit
Lunch	3–4 servings	45–60 g	Meat sandwich with two slices of bread, 8 oz. milk, 1/2c canned fruit (water packed). Vegetable salad/w dressing
Midafternoon snack	1–2 servings	15–30 g	Half cheese sandwich, 8 oz. milk
Supper	3–4 servings	45–60 grams	Roast beef, green beans, 2/3c rice, dinner roll, small fresh fruit, unsweetened beverage
HS snack	1–2 servings	15–30 g	Half meat sandwich, light yogurt

GDM diet has approximately 2200–2400 calories when snacks are included

9.7   Criteria to Begin Concurrent Therapy

- In patients compliant with diet, when 20% of all blood glucose values are above glycemic goals, medication should be initiated.
- Be aware of patients who achieve euglycemia by severe calorie restriction as evidenced by weight loss and ketones in the urine. In these patients encourage an appropriate diet and medication.

9.8   Treatment of Hypoglycemia (Rule of 15)

- Assess reason for hypoglycemia.
- Rule of 15: Take 15 grams of carbohydrate every 15 min until blood glucose reaches 100.
- 15 grams = 1/2c orange juice, five to six Life Savers candy, 8 oz. glass of milk, four glucose tablets, and four to six crackers.

References

1. Han S, Middleton P, Shepherd E, Van Ryswyk E, Crowther CA. Different types of dietary advice for women with gestational diabetes mellitus. Cochrane Database Syst Rev. 2017;2:CD009275. doi:10.1002/14651858.CD009275.pub3.
2. Pope E, Koren G, Bozzo P. Sugar substitutes during pregnancy. Can Fam Physician. 2014;60(11):1003–5.
3. Committee on Practice Bulletins—Obstetrics. Practice bulletin no. 137: gestational diabetes mellitus. Obstet Gynecol. 2013; 122(2 Pt 1):406–16. doi:10.1097/01.AOG.0000433006.09219.f1.
4. Kaiser L, Allen LH, American Dietetic Association. Position of the American dietetic association: nutrition and lifestyle for a healthy pregnancy outcome. J Am Diet Assoc. 2008;108(3): 553–61.
5. Goodnight W, Newman R. Society of maternal-fetal M. Optimal nutrition for improved twin pregnancy outcome. Obstet Gynecol. 2009;114(5):1121–34. doi:10.1097/AOG.0b013e3181bb14c8.

6. Hernandez TL. Carbohydrate content in the GDM diet: two views: view 1: nutrition therapy in gestational diabetes: the case for complex carbohydrates. Diabetes Spectrum. 2016;29(2):82–8. doi:10.2337/diaspect.29.2.82.
7. Hernandez TL, Van Pelt RE, Anderson MA, Reece MS, Reynolds RM, de la Houssaye BA, Heerwagen M, Donahoo WT, Daniels LJ, Chartier-Logan C, Janssen RC, Friedman JE, Barbour LA. Women with gestational diabetes mellitus randomized to a higher-complex carbohydrate/low-fat diet manifest lower adipose tissue insulin resistance, inflammation, glucose, and free fatty acids: a pilot study. Diabetes Care. 2016;39(1):39–42. doi:10.2337/dc15-0515.

Chapter 10
Insulin

Lisa E. Moore

Fast Facts

- Insulin cannot be taken orally but it can be inhaled.
- All insulin sold in the United States is manufactured in a laboratory.
- Although insulin is excreted in breast milk, its protein structure is destroyed in the digestive tract.
- Insulin does not cross the placenta.

10.1 Introduction

Human insulin is a dimeric polypeptide chain of 50 amino acids. The basic structure of insulin is conserved across species, and humans are able to use insulin from nonhuman sources. Porcine insulin differs from human insulin by only a single amino acid. Insulin is considered an essential medication by the World Health Organization.

L.E. Moore, MD, FACOG
Department of Obstetrics and Gynecology, Texas Tech University Health Sciences Center El Paso, Paul L. Foster School of Medicine, El Paso, TX, USA
e-mail: lisa.e.moore@ttuhsc.edu

© Springer International Publishing AG 2018
L.E. Moore (ed.), *Diabetes in Pregnancy*,
https://doi.org/10.1007/978-3-319-65518-5_10

Insulin is secreted from the beta cells of the pancreas as proinsulin. The proinsulin molecule is cleaved to produce C-peptide and mature insulin. Synthetic human insulin is made by inserting the gene for human insulin into bacteria or yeast.

10.2   Descriptive Qualities of Insulin

All types of insulin are described by three aspects of time: onset, peak, and duration:

- Onset is the length of time after injection that it takes insulin to reach the bloodstream and start to affect blood glucose levels.
- Peak is the length of time after injection that the action of the insulin is at its highest level.
- Duration is the length of time after injection that insulin will continue to lower blood glucose.

Insulin is also described by its strength or the number of units of insulin per milliliter:

- U100 is the most commonly used strength in the United States. 1 mL of U100 insulin contains 100 units of insulin.
- U500 is also available but less commonly used. 1 mL of U500 insulin contains 500 units of insulin.
- U100 is typically dispensed as a 10 mL vial or 100 units of insulin. U500 is dispensed as a 20 mL vial which contains 10,000 units of insulin.

10.3   Storage of Insulin

Unopened bottles and pens of insulin should be stored in the refrigerator. If kept at 36–46 F, insulin is good up to the expiration date. If kept at room temperature 56–80 F, insulin will last approximately 28 days. Higher temperatures may shorten the time. Insulin will also become less effective over time when stored at room temperature. Cold insulin may be painful to inject.

10.4   Initiation of Insulin

Insulin dosing for marked hyperglycemia should be based on current weight and gestational age. The gestational age matters because insulin resistance is expected to increase as the pregnancy progresses and the placenta grows.

Total daily starting doses can be calculated using the tables below:

Total daily starting dose: method 1 (adapted from Jovanovic, Clin Obstet Gynecol. 2000)

0.7 U/kg	From 1 to 18 weeks
0.8 U/kg	From 18 to 26 weeks
0.9 U/kg	From 26 to 36 weeks
1.0 U/kg	>36 weeks

Total daily starting dose: method 2

First trimester	0.7 U/kg
Second trimester	0.8 U/kg
Third trimester	0.9–1.0 U/kg

For patients with hyperglycemia, throughout the day both at fasting and with meals, start insulin using a combination of rapid-acting insulin with meals and an intermediate-acting insulin to cover between meals and fasting in the morning.

10.4.1   Quick-Start Method #1

Total daily dose = (weight in kg x TDD(c))/4 where TDD(c) is the constant based on gestational age.

Example: 86 kg woman at 25 weeks
86 × 0.8 = 68.8
68.8/4 = 17.2
Give 17 units of rapid-acting insulin (aspart or Humalog) 15 min before each meal and 17 units of NPH at night.

Patients with type 1 IDDM and patients with hyperglycemia between meals can use Lantus (same dose) instead of NPH.

10.4.2   Method #2

Calculate the total daily dose as in method #1	68.8 (round to 69)
Divide the TDD by 3 (into 3rds)	1/3 = 23; 2/3 = 46
Divide the 2/3 into 3rds which will be given in am	46/3 = 15; 1/3 = 15; 2/3 = 30
For the morning give 1/3 rapid acting and 2/3 intermediate	15u aspart and 30 U NPH in am
Divide the remaining 1/3 by 2 (into half)	15/2 = 7.5 (round up to 8)
Give half as rapid-acting insulin before dinner	8 U of aspart before dinner
Give half as intermediate-acting insulin before bedtime	8 U of NPH at bedtime

It has been my experience that these methods of calculating dosage are equivalent in efficacy.

10.4.3   Fasting Hyperglycemia

Persistent fasting hyperglycemia mild >95 mg/dl <120 mg/dl:

- Give 0.1 units/kg of NPH at bedtime, increase as needed, or use weight-based dosing.
- Note—this degree of hyperglycemia may be treatable with oral agents.

Persistent fasting hyperglycemia moderate to severe >120 mg/dl:

- Give 0.2–0.25 units/kg of NPH at bedtime, increase as needed, or use weight-based dosing.

10.4.4   Postprandial Hyperglycemia

One hour after meals >140 mg/dl <180 mg/dl:

- Give 0.2 units/kg of aspart or lispro 15 min before meals or calculate weight-based dose.

One hour after meals >180 mg/dl:

- Weight-based dose of aspart or lispro before meals— increase as needed.
- Review diet.
- If lunch is high, consider adding NPH at breakfast (eat lunch 4–5 h after breakfast).
- If dinner is high, adjust premeal aspart or lispro.

10.4.5   Hypoglycemia (≤60 mg/dl)

Fasting or during the night, decrease bed time NPH by 2–5 units.
After meals decrease mealtime aspart or lispro by 2 units and review diet.

10.4.6   A Few Key Points

- A calculated starting dose is only a starting point and adjustment will be required.
- As the pregnancy progresses, insulin requirement will increase.
- Insulin should not be adjusted for random excursions— modify dosing when there is a consistent pattern.
- Patients on insulin must still follow a diet and count carbohydrates.
- Regular moderate exercise can reduce the insulin requirement.

10.4.7   Alphabetized List of Selected Insulins and Injectables

See Table 10.1 for quick reference.

Table 10.1 Common insulins and non-insulin injectables

Insulin	Onset	Peak	Duration	Pregnancy	Lactation	Notes
Rapid acting						
Aspart (NovoLog)	<15 m	30–90 m	3–5 h	+	+	
Lispro (Humalog)	<15 m	30–90 m	3–5 h	+	+	
Glulisine (Apidra)	<15 m	30–90 m	3–5 h	+	+	
Afrezza				+	+	
Short acting						
Regular	<1 h	2–4 h	4–8 h	+	+	Clear
Intermediate acting						
NPH	1–2 h	4–10 h	10–18 h	+	+	Cloudy
Peakless/long acting						
Glargine (Lantus)	1–2 h	NA	24 h	+	+	Do not mix
Detemir (Levemir)	1–2 h	NA	24 h	+	+	

Ultralong acting						
Degludec (Tresiba)	30–90 m	NA	42 h	+	+	
Combinations						
50:50 NPH:Lispro	2 h/15 m	≤10 h/1.5 h	≤18 h/5 h	+	+	
75:25 NPH: Lispro	2 h/15 m	≤10 h/1.5 h	≤18 h/5 h	+	+	
70:30 NPH: Regular	2 h/1 h	≤10 h/4 h	≤18 h/8 h	+	+	
Non-insulin injectables GLP-1 agonists						
Dulaglutide (Trulicity)	—	—	7 d	—	—	Not studied in pregnancy
Exenatide (Byetta)	—	—	12 h	—	—	Not studied in pregnancy
Liraglutide (Victoza)	—	—	24 h	—	—	Not studied in pregnancy

10.5   Afrezza: Recombinant (*E. coli*) Inhaled Regular Insulin Delivered by Nebulizer

Onset 15–20 min; peak 1 h; duration 2–3 h
   Available in three strengths: 4 units (blue), 8 units (green), 12 units (yellow) (www.afrezza.com)

10.5.1   Pregnancy

Afrezza has not been studied in pregnancy and should not be used unless the potential benefit justifies potential risk to the fetus (formerly FDA pregnancy category C).
   In rats given the carrier molecule at doses of 30 mg, 60 mg, and 100 mg/kg, no major malformations were observed.
   In rabbits given 30 mg, 60 mg, and 100 mg per kg of body, adverse maternal effects were seen at all doses in breastfeeding.
   Both the insulin and the carrier molecule are found in breast milk.

10.5.2   Precautions

Co-administration with albuterol increases the amount of insulin absorbed.

10.6   Aspart (NovoLog): Recombinant (Baker's Yeast), Homologous to Human Insulin Except a Single Amino Acid

Onset 20 min; peak 1–3 h; duration 3–5 h
   Available as 10 mL vial (U100); 3 mL Penfill cartridges; 3 mL FlexPen; 3 mL FlexTouch (www.novologpro.com)

10.6.1   Pregnancy

Studies in animals do not demonstrate a risk to the fetus.

Case series available in human pregnancy with no adverse effects.

No controlled studies in human pregnancy (FDA pregnancy category B).

10.6.2   Breastfeeding

Safe in breastfeeding

10.7   Degludec (Tresiba) Recombinant (Baker's Yeast)

Onset 30–90 min; no peak; duration >24 h

Available as 3 mL prefilled FlexPen (u200, u100) (www. tresiba.com)

10.7.1   Pregnancy

Rats and rabbits were exposed to insulin degludec in animal reproduction studies during organogenesis.

Pre- and postimplantation losses and visceral/skeletal abnormalities were observed in rats at doses five times (rat) and at ten times (rabbit) the human exposure at a dose of 0.75 U/kg/day.

These effects were similar to those observed in rats administered human insulin (NPH).

FDA pregnancy category C.

10.7.2   Breastfeeding

Studies in rats have shown insulin degludec is secreted in rat milk in a concentration that is lower than in plasma. No adverse effects are anticipated in breastfed infants due to destruction of the molecule in the digestive tract.

10.7.3   Precautions

Do not mix with other insulins or solutions.

10.8   Detemir (Levemir) Recombinant (Baker's Yeast) Clear

Onset 1–2 h; no peak; duration 24 h
    Available as 10 mL vial (u100) FlexTouch pen 3 mL (u100) (www.levemir.com)

10.8.1   Pregnancy

Pregnancy category—does not cross the placenta

10.8.2   Breastfeeding

Safe in breastfeeding

10.9   Glargine (Lantus, Basaglar, Toujeo): Recombinant (*E. coli*) Lantus Is a Clear Long-Acting Insulin

Onset 1–2 h; no peak; duration 20–24 h
    Available as 10 mL vial (u100); SoloSTAR pen 3 mL (u100) (www.lantus.com)

10.9.1   Pregnancy

Animal studies in pregnancy do not show an increased risk to the fetus.

Case series available in human pregnancy with no adverse effects.

10.9.2   Breastfeeding

Safe in breastfeeding

10.9.3   Precautions

Do not mix with other insulins.

10.10   Glulisine (Apidra): Recombinant (*E. coli*), Equipotent to Human Insulin with Quicker Onset and Shorter Duration

Dose 15 min before meals or within 20 min of starting a meal
   Onset 15 min; peak 1 h; duration 2–4 h
   Available as 10 mL vial (U100) or 3 mL SoloSTAR prefilled pen (www.apidra.com)

10.10.1   Pregnancy

Pregnant animals received subcutaneous doses up to 10 units/kg once daily (an exposure two times the average human dose based on body surface area comparison), and no toxic effect was noted on embryo-fetal development. Adverse effects on embryo-fetal development were only seen at maternal toxic dose levels inducing hypoglycemia. There are no controlled data in human pregnancy (formerly pregnancy category C).

10.10.2   Breastfeeding

Safe in breast feeding

10.11   Lispro (Humalog) Recombinant (*E. coli*)

Onset 15–20 min; peak 1–3 h; duration 3–5 h
   Available as 10 mL vial (u100) KwikPen 3 mL (u100, u200) (www.humalog.com)

10.11.1   Pregnancy

Safe in pregnancy—extensive history of use in pregnancy (FDA category B)

10.11.2   Breastfeeding

Safe in breastfeeding
NPH (Novolin N; Humulin N) cloudy
Onset 2 h; peak 4–12 h; duration 18–26 h
Available as 10 mL vial (u100). KwikPen 3 mL (u100)

10.11.3   Pregnancy

Safe in pregnancy—does not cross the placenta

10.11.4   Breastfeeding

Safe in breastfeeding
   Regular (Novolin R and Humulin R) Novolin is recombinant from Baker's yeast and Humulin from *E. coli*.
   Onset 30 min; peak 1–3 h; duration 6–8 h
   Available in 10 mL (u100) or 20 mL vial (u500); KwikPen 3 mL (u100)

10.11.5   Pregnancy

Safe in pregnancy—does not cross the placenta

10.11.6 Breastfeeding

Safe in breastfeeding

10.11.7 Non-insulin Injectables

All drugs in this category are GLP-1 agonists.

GLP-1 is a hormone that is secreted by cells in the ileum based on the presence of food in the lumen of the small intestine. GLP-1 induces beta cells to release insulin and at the same time suppresses glucagon secretion.

All drugs in this category have been associated with the development of thyroid C-cell tumors at clinically relevant exposures in both genders of rats and mice. It is not known if the use of these drugs is associated with thyroid C-cell tumors in humans.

GLP-1 agonist should not be used in patients with type 1 diabetes.

10.12 Dulaglutide (Trulicity)

Once weekly injection

Supplied as single-dose prefilled pens or prefilled syringes: 0.75 mg/0.5 mL; 1.5 mg/0.5 mL (www.trulicity.com)

10.12.1 Pregnancy

There are no adequate and well-controlled studies in pregnant women. Studies in animals show fetal growth reductions and ossification defects (formerly pregnancy category C).

10.12.2 Breastfeeding

It is unknown whether Trulicity is excreted in human breast milk and cessation of the drug during breastfeeding should be considered.

10.13   Exenatide (Byetta, Bydureon, Saxenda)

Twice daily injection
Supplied in prefilled multidose pens 250 mcg/mL: pens available as 1.2 mL pen with 60 doses of 5 mcg each or 2.4 mL pen with 60 doses of 10 mcg each (www.byetta.com; www.bydureon.com)

10.13.1   Pregnancy

Studies in animals demonstrate an association with irregular skeletal ossification defects, cleft palate, and neonatal death. There are no studies in pregnant women.
A registry for patient exposed to Exenatide during pregnancy has been implemented, and exposed patients or their providers are encouraged to participate.

10.13.2   Breastfeeding

To date it is not known if Exenatide is excreted in human breast milk. In animals the amount in breast milk is less than or equal to 2.5% of plasma levels.

10.14   Liraglutide (Victoza)

Once daily injection
Supplied in prefilled multidose pens containing 6 mg/mL. Doses of 0.6 mg, 1.2 mg, or 1.8 mg (www.victoza.com)

10.14.1   Pregnancy

In animals there was an increased risk of miscarriage and of minor skeletal defects, growth restriction, and visceral abnormalities. There are no human studies.

10.14.2   Breastfeeding

Breastfeeding is not recommended. In rats, concentrations approaching 50% of the maternal plasma level were found in breast milk.

10.15   Summary

NPH, regular insulin, Lantus, detemir, and the short-acting analogues lispro and aspart have been extensively used during pregnancy and are considered safe. Insulin is excreted in breast milk, but its protein structure is destroyed by digestive enzymes. The GLP-1 agonists have not been studied in pregnancy.

References

1. Jovanovic L. Role of diet and insulin treatment of diabetes in pregnancy. Clin Obstet Gynecol. 2000;43(1):46–55.
2. www.afrezza.com
3. www.novologpro.com
4. www.tresiba.com
5. www.levemir.com
6. www.lantus.com
7. www.apidra.com
8. www.humalog.com
9. www.trulicity.com
10. www.byetta.com
11. www.bydureon.com
12. www.victoza.com

Chapter 11
Oral Hypoglycemic Agents

Lisa E. Moore

> **Fast Facts**
>
> - A systematic review found no difference in maternal or neonatal outcomes when either glyburide or metformin was compared to insulin in women with GDM [1].
> - Insulin and oral agents are equivalent in efficacy, and either can be used as first-line therapy in women with GDM according to ACOG practice bulletin 137 [2].

11.1 Introduction

Glyburide and metformin are the two most commonly used oral agents for management of diabetes during pregnancy. Acarbose has been studied in pregnancy but is less often used than the other two agents. Although insulin is still considered

L.E. Moore, MD, FACOG
Department of Obstetrics and Gynecology, Texas Tech University Health Sciences Center El Paso, Paul L. Foster School of Medicine, El Paso, TX, USA
e-mail: lisa.e.moore@ttuhsc.edu

© Springer International Publishing AG 2018
L.E. Moore (ed.), *Diabetes in Pregnancy*,
https://doi.org/10.1007/978-3-319-65518-5_11

the gold standard for treatment of diabetes requiring medication, there is compelling evidence that oral agents provide equivalent glycemic control and maternal and neonatal outcomes when compared to insulin in patients with gestational diabetes. Additionally, the use of oral agents enhances compliance by ease of use and is cost-effective. Table 11.1 provides an overview of the oral agents currently used in pregnancy.

11.2   Glyburide

Glyburide is a second-generation sulfonylurea that works by stimulating the pancreas to release insulin. It is FDA pregnancy category B and is also considered safe during breastfeeding. The drug comes in 1.25, 2.5, and 5 mg tablets. The peak onset of action is at 4 h. Glyburide may have low but detectable levels in the blood up to 24 h after dosing. There is also a micronized version of the drug which has not been studied in pregnancy. Starting dose is either 1.25 mg or 2.5 mg once or twice a day based on blood glucose. The maximum dose is 20 mg a day.

In 2000 Langer published his landmark study comparing pregnant women with gestational diabetes randomized to either glyburide or insulin. There was no difference in glycemic control or in neonatal outcomes. Four percent of patients on glyburide failed to meet glycemic goals and required insulin. Hypoglycemic episodes, defined as blood glucose <40 mg/dL, occurred in 20% of the patients on insulin compared to only 4% of the glyburide patients. Cord blood was collected at delivery simultaneously with maternal serum. No neonates had measureable levels of glyburide in the cord blood although glyburide was detected in the maternal blood [3].

In a retrospective cohort of women on insulin compared to women on glyburide, there were no differences in birth weight or the incidence of large for gestational age infants. The patients on glyburide had a higher incidence of preeclampsia and hyperbilirubinemia in the infants. Babies of women in the insulin group were more likely to be admitted to the NICU [4].

TABLE 11.1 Oral agents used in pregnancy

	Glyburide	Metformin	Acarbose	Glucovance
Supplied as	1.25, 2.5, 5 mg	500, 850, 1000 mg	25, 50, 100 mg	1.25/250, 2.5/500, 5/500 mg
Starting dose	1.25–2.5 mg QD or BID	500 mg QD or BID	25 mg TID with meals	1.25/250 mg
Maximum dose	20 mg/day	2000 mg/day	50 mg TID <60 kg 100 mg TID >60 kg	20/2000 mg/day
Peak serum level	4 h	1–3 h	1 h	1–3 h
Side effects	Nausea, vomiting Pruritic rash, hypoglycemia	GI upset	GI upset	Same as metformin and glyburide
Contraindications	Sulfa allergy G6PD deficiency	Renal disease Liver disease	Bowel obstruction Chronic constipation	

Glyburide should not be used in women with a sulfa allergy. Patients with G6PD deficiency may develop hemolytic anemia.

Side effects of glyburide include nausea, vomiting, diarrhea, and a pruritic rash. The most commonly reported side effect is hypoglycemia.

11.3   Metformin

Metformin works by inhibiting gluconeogenesis and decreasing peripheral resistance to insulin. It is cleared by the kidneys and excreted in urine. Metformin immediate release comes in 500, 850, and 1000 mg tablets. A generic form is available. Metformin slow release (SR) or extended release (XR) is available in 500, 700, and 1000 mg tablets. The peak onset of action is from 1 to 3 h after taking the immediate release form and within 4–8 h with the extended release formulation. The starting dose is 500 mg which can be given once or twice a day. The maximum dose is 2000 mg a day.

Side effects include GI upset with flatulence and diarrhea. The GI side effects tend to resolve within a week of use. Metformin carries a black box warning about the risk of lactic acidosis. The risk of lactic acidosis is increased in patient with kidney or liver disease and with high alcohol intake.

Metformin is FDA pregnancy category B and is considered safe in breastfeeding. Metformin has been shown to cross the placenta in appreciable amounts. The concentration of metformin that reaches the fetus may be similar to maternal concentrations.

In a study of women randomized to metformin or insulin, neonatal hypoglycemia was less common in the metformin group; otherwise neonatal outcomes were not different. A hypothesis of the study was that metformin exposure in utero would be associated with less insulin resistance and central fat in the offspring. At 2 years of age, in comparison to the insulin group, there was no difference in central fat measures, total fat mass, or percentage of body fat [5].

Babies of women who conceived on metformin while being treated for PCOS and continued the drug during pregnancy were followed for 18 months. There were no fetal anomalies. Height and weight were compared at 3, 6, 9, and 12 months to data from the Center for Disease Control and Prevention. Males were shorter at 3 months in the metformin group. Females were shorter at birth than CDC controls and shorter and thinner at 3 months but matched in size by 6 months. No infants were found to have motor or social delay when evaluated using the American Academy of Pediatrics motor-social development questionnaire [6].

The Metformin in Gestational Diabetes (MiG) trial is the largest to date to study metformin to insulin. Three hundred and sixty-three women were randomized to metformin, and 370 were randomized to insulin. 46.3% of the women on metformin required supplemental insulin. In a smaller study comparing metformin to glyburide, metformin had twice the failure rate of glyburide. Neonatal outcomes were similar [7].

The MiG study also looked at the convenience of metformin use by administering a questionnaire to patients at 1 week postpartum. 76.6% of women would choose metformin in a subsequent pregnancy compared to 27% of women who would choose insulin again.

Metformin has a high failure rate when used as a single agent to manage GDM. In a randomized trial comparing metformin to glyburide, the failure rate to control blood glucose was twice as high for metformin [8]. In a study comparing metformin to insulin, 46.3% of patients on metformin alone required the additional insulin [7, 9].

11.4 Glucovance

Glucovance is a combination drug containing metformin and glyburide. It is FDA pregnancy category B. The drug is available in 1.25/250, 2.5/500, and 5/500 mg doses. The starting dose is 1.25/250 once a day for drug-naïve patients due to the risk of hypoglycemia. Contraindications to use are those associated with both glyburide and metformin use. There are no studies of Glucovance use in pregnancy.

11.5   Acarbose

Acarbose inhibits the action of alpha-glucosidase in the brush border of the small intestine and the action of pancreatic alpha-amylase. The net effect is to limit the ability to digest complex carbohydrates. Side effects of acarbose are those associated with delivery of undigested carbohydrates to the colon and include flatulence and diarrhea. Side effects are dose related. Acarbose is FDA pregnancy category B. Acarbose is supplied as 25, 50, and 100 mg tablets. There is no fixed dosing regimen. Acarbose should be taken three times a day with the first bite of each meal. The maximum dose per day is 100 mg TID for patients >60 kg and 50 mg TID for patients <60 kg. It is recommended to start at the smallest dose both to reduce the gastrointestinal side effects and to avoid hypoglycemia. To treat hypoglycemia due to acarbose use liquid glucose or glucose tablets. Sucrose (table sugar) won't work due to the action of the drug.

Zarate treated six women with GDM with acarbose. They normalized their blood glucose but experienced gastrointestinal symptoms for the entire course of treatment [10].

In an open randomized trial of insulin, glyburide, and acarbose in women with gestational diabetes, 42% of patients on acarbose were not adequately controlled compared to 20.8% of patients on glyburide [11].

In a study comparing metformin and acarbose for ovulation induction in women with polycystic ovarian syndrome, the rate of flatulence and/or diarrhea was higher in metformin than in acarbose. Patients on metformin had a significant decrease in BMI and fasting blood glucose compared to those on acarbose [12].

11.6   Summary

Metformin and glyburide have been well studied in pregnancy and are considered safe. Acarbose has not been as well studied but may also be an option for treating diabetes in pregnancy.

References

1. Nicholson W, Bolen S, Witkop CT, Neale D, Wilson L, Bass E. Benefits and risks of oral diabetes agents compared with insulin in women with gestational diabetes: a systematic review. Obstet Gynecol. 2009;113(1):193–205. doi:10.1097/AOG.0b013e318190a459.
2. Committee on Practice B-O. Practice bulletin no. 137: gestational diabetes mellitus. Obstet Gynecol. 2013;122(2 Pt 1):406–16. doi:10.1097/01.AOG.0000433006.09219.f1.
3. Langer O, Conway DL, Berkus MD, Xenakis EM, Gonzales O. A comparison of glyburide and insulin in women with gestational diabetes mellitus. N Engl J Med. 2000;343(16):1134–8. doi:10.1056/NEJM200010193431601.
4. Jacobson GF, Ramos GA, Ching JY, Kirby RS, Ferrara A, Field DR. Comparison of glyburide and insulin for the management of gestational diabetes in a large managed care organization. Am J Obstet Gynecol. 2005;193(1):118–24. doi:10.1016/j.ajog.2005.03.018.
5. Rowan JA, Rush EC, Obolonkin V, Battin M, Wouldes T, Hague WM. Metformin in gestational diabetes: the offspring follow-up (MiG TOFU): body composition at 2 years of age. Diabetes Care. 2011;34(10):2279–84. doi:10.2337/dc11-0660.
6. Glueck CJ, Goldenberg N, Pranikoff J, Loftspring M, Sieve L, Wang P. Height, weight, and motor-social development during the first 18 months of life in 126 infants born to 109 mothers with polycystic ovary syndrome who conceived on and continued metformin through pregnancy. Hum Reprod. 2004;19(6):1323–30. doi:10.1093/humrep/deh263.
7. Rowan JA, Hague WM, Gao W, Battin MR, Moore MP, Mi GTI. Metformin versus insulin for the treatment of gestational

diabetes. N Engl J Med. 2008;358(19):2003–15. doi:10.1056/NEJMoa0707193.

8. Moore LE, Clokey D, Rappaport VJ, Curet LB. Metformin compared with glyburide in gestational diabetes: a randomized controlled trial. Obstet Gynecol. 2010;115(1):55–9. doi:10.1097/AOG.0b013e3181c52132.

9. Rowan JA, Mi GI. A trial in progress: gestational diabetes. Treatment with metformin compared with insulin (the metformin in gestational diabetes [MiG] trial). Diabetes Care. 2007;30(Suppl 2):S214–9. doi:10.2337/dc07-s219.

10. Zarate A, Ochoa R, Hernandez M, Basurto L. Effectiveness of acarbose in the control of glucose tolerance worsening in pregnancy. Ginecol Obstet Mex. 2000;68:42–5.

11. Bertini AM, Silva JC, Taborda W, Becker F, Lemos Bebber FR, Zucco Viesi JM, Aquim G, Ribeiro TE. Perinatal outcomes and the use of oral hypoglycemic agents. J Perinat Med. 2005;33(6):519–23. doi:10.1515/JPM.2005.092.

12. Hanjalic-Beck A, Gabriel B, Schaefer W, Zahradnik HP, Schories M, Tempfer C, Keck C, Denschlag D. Metformin versus acarbose therapy in patients with polycystic ovary syndrome (PCOS): a prospective randomised double-blind study. Gynecol Endocrinol. 2010;26(9):690–7. doi:10.3109/09513591003686379.

Chapter 12
Basic Insulin Pump Management

Lisa E. Moore

> **Fast Facts**
>
> - Insulin pumps typically use only rapid-acting insulin.
> - Pump infusion sites should be rotated every 48 h during pregnancy.
> - Unless the pump incorporates glucose monitoring, the patient will still have to check blood glucose four to six times each day.

12.1 Introduction

The insulin pump or the continuous subcutaneous insulin infusion (CSII) was developed to provide insulin in a manner resembling the physiologic availability of insulin. Indications for using an insulin pump essentially include any patient unable to achieve adequate glucose control in the setting of patient compliance. Patients receiving insulin injections who

L.E. Moore, MD, FACOG
Department of Obstetrics and Gynecology, Texas Tech University
Health Sciences Center El Paso, Paul L. Foster School of Medicine,
El Paso, TX, USA
e-mail: lisa.e.moore@ttuhsc.edu

© Springer International Publishing AG 2018
L.E. Moore (ed.), *Diabetes in Pregnancy*,
https://doi.org/10.1007/978-3-319-65518-5_12

do not achieve euglycemia due to noncompliance with diet and self-monitoring will not, in general, improve on an insulin pump. The American Association of Clinical Endocrinologists has defined criteria for patients who are not good candidates for the pump as listed in Box 1 [1]. For compliant patients the benefits of a pump include better control, fewer and less severe hypoglycemic episodes, and normalization of lifestyle. Complications of the pump include lipohypertrophy at infusion sites, rashes and skin infections at the infusion site, and pump failure resulting in hyperglycemia.

Few studies have looked at the use of the insulin pump during pregnancy. The available studies do not show a difference in outcomes between women on the insulin pump compared to women taking multiple daily doses of insulin to control blood glucose during pregnancy [2, 3].

Very few medical professionals have experience or knowledge about the insulin pump. The insulin pump is a complex medical device which, used incorrectly, can result in significant morbidity and mortality. Extensive training is required for managing the insulin pump. This chapter is intended to provide an overview of pump management and a knowledge base for providers caring for patients on the pump.

Box 1: Characteristics of Patients Who are Not Good Candidates for the Insulin Pump

- Unwilling or unable to perform multiple daily injections, regular self-monitoring of blood glucose, and carbohydrate counting
- Lack of motivation and/or a history of nonadherence to prescribed insulin regimens
- History of serious psychological or psychiatric conditions
- Unwilling to accept limitations of pump therapy (e.g., the belief that using the pump will eliminate the need to follow diet)

12.2   Pump Basics

Pregnant patients usually present already on the pump, and it falls to the provider to adjust the pump settings. Transitioning to using the pump is not recommended during pregnancy because it can take up to 3 months to become comfortable with using the pump and to achieve glycemic control.

An insulin pump provides insulin in two ways:

Bolus insulin is insulin delivered "on demand" to correct blood glucose levels or to compensate for food intake.

Basal insulin is a continuous infusion of insulin that is ongoing 24 h a day and mimics the function of the pancreas. Basal insulin maintains euglycemia between meals.

The total daily dose (TDD) is the basal + bolus insulin used each day.

12.2.1   Pump TDD

The pump TDD can be calculated by three methods [1]:

Method 1:

Reduce the daily dose of pre-pump insulin by 25%:

$$TDD \times 0.75 = \text{the reduced daily dose}$$

Method 2:

Calculate based on weight:

$$\text{Weight in kg} \times 0.5 \text{ u} = \text{the weight-based dose}$$

Method 3:

Take the average of weight-based dosing and the reduced daily dose:

$$\text{Pump TDD} = \left(\text{weight-based dose} + \text{reduced daily dose}\right) / 2$$

Example: An 85 kg patient takes 15 units of aspart with each meal and 15 units of NPH at bedtime.

$$\text{Pump TDD} = 85(0.5) + 60(0.75)/2 = 43.75\,\text{u}/\text{day}$$

Next calculate how much to give as basal insulin and how much as bolus.

12.2.2   Basal Insulin

For adults, 40–50% should be basal insulin and the remainder should be bolus. A 50/50 split between bolus and basal is a reasonable starting point. As with all diabetes management, the initial dosing can be modified as needed.

The basal rate is then divided into the amount to be given each hour for 24 h.

Example:
The pump TDD = 43.75 u/day
The basal rate = 43.75 × 0.5 = 21.9 u/day then the hourly rate = 21.9/24 = 0.9 u/h
The daily total bolus should be 43.75 × 0.5 = 21.9 u/day
This number is divided by 3 to give a fixed amount of bolus insulin with each meal. 21.9/3 = 7.3 u with each meal

Another method is to use a weight-based calculation of the basal rate and to set four individual basal rates based on diurnal variation. To use this method, calculate the total basal amount at 0.2–0.4 × weight in kg. The following schedules can be used as a start. Time periods can be individualized as needed.

A. Midnight to 4 am (4 h) 0.1 × basal—covers nighttime blood glucose
B. 4–8 am (4 h) 0.2 × basal—covers fasting blood glucose
C. 8 am to 4 pm (8 h) 0.3 × basal—daytime between meal coverage
D. 4 pm to midnight (8 h) 0.4 × basal—evening and bedtime coverage

Example: 70 kg woman
Basal insulin = 0.3 × 70 = 21 u/day
A = 0.1 × 21 = 2.1 u over 4 h = 0.5 u/h
B = 0.2 × 21 = 4.2 u over 4 h = 1.1 u/h
C = 0.3 × 21 = 6.3 u over 8 h = 0.78 u/h
D = 0.4 × 21 = 8.4 u over 8 h = 1.1 u/h

Adjustments to the basal rate(s) should be made in 0.1–0.3 u increments. As you can see having four schedules allows individualized adjustments based on patients actual blood glucose during that time.

A couple of facts should be kept in mind: In the mornings due to gluconeogenesis, blood glucose levels tend to rise (dawn phenomenon). This is covered by schedule B. During the day physical activity helps to keep blood glucose lower so schedule C may be lower also. Evening to bedtime is usually another time of reduced activity with a higher basal rate. However, exceptions, such as a patient who exercises for an hour after work each day, should be taken into account. Episodes of hypoglycemia are more common during midnight to 4am period (schedule A).

12.2.3   Premeal Bolus Insulin

Premeal insulin can be a bolus of a fixed amount or it can be calculated for each meal.

To calculate bolus dosing with meals, two numbers are needed, the insulin correction factor (ICF) and the insulin-to-carbohydrate ratio (ICR).

12.3   The Insulin Correction Factor

The insulin correction factor also known as the insulin sensitivity factor is the number of mg/dl that one unit of insulin will lower the blood glucose. This number is used to calculate how much bolus insulin to give.

Many patients will already know their insulin correction factor. If not, the rule of 1700 can be used to calculate the correction factor. Actually numbers between 1600 and 2200 are used to calculate the ICF. The higher the number, the greater the anticipated point drop from a unit of insulin (i.e. the more sensitive to insulin effect).

The Rule of 1700 and 2000
1700/pump TDD = ICF or
2000/pump TDD = ICF

To calculate the amount of corrective insulin required to compensate for the current blood glucose, use the following formula:

$$(\text{Blood glucose} - \text{target glucose}) / \text{ICF}$$

Notice that this will be a negative number if the blood glucose is below target:

Target = 95 mg/dL; ICF = 30 mg/dL

Example 1: Blood glucose is 150 mg/dL
(150–95)/30 = 1.8 units (add 1.8 units to the bolus dose).
Example 2: Blood glucose is 65 mg/dL
(65–95)/30 = −1 units (subtract 1 unit from the bolus dose).

The insulin-to-carbohydrate ratio (ICR) tells you how many grams of carbohydrate are covered by one unit of insulin.

The ICR is calculated using the rule of 450:

450/Pump TDD = ICR

> Example: Pump TDD = 50 u/day
> ICR = 450/50 = 9 g/u of insulin

Use the ICR to compensate for the carbohydrate in an upcoming meal.

> Example: You are at a fast-food restaurant and you are planning to eat the super duper burger with fries and a drink. Calorie and carbohydrate values are conveniently displayed, and your planned meal contains 154 g of carbohydrate. ICR = 9 g/u.
> 154/9 = 17 u of insulin to cover this meal

There is one more step to calculating the amount of bolus insulin to give for this meal.

Note that prior to the meal, you checked your blood glucose and used that value to calculate the amount of insulin needed to correct if you were high or low.

The amount of bolus insulin is equal to the corrective insulin plus the compensatory insulin for the meal.

> Example: ICF = 30 mg/dL; ICR = 9 g/u
> Target glucose is 95 mg/dL and your current glucose is 65 mg/dL corrective insulin = −1 units.
> Planned meal contains 154 g of carbohydrates compensatory insulin = 17 u.
> Bolus for this meal = 16 units of insulin.

All insulin pumps now have a bolus insulin calculation feature (a wizard). The ICR and ICF are entered into the pump settings. It is necessary to enter the premeal blood glucose measurement, and the amount of carbohydrates in the upcoming meal and the amount of bolus are calculated.

Bolus insulin can be delivered in different ways depending on the type of pump:

- Standard bolus: All of the bolus insulin is delivered at one time prior to the meal.
- Delayed bolus (extended, square wave): Bolus is infused slowly over several hours.
- Combination (multi-wave, dual wave): Part of the bolus is delivered at the start of the meal, and the rest is infused over several hours.

12.4   Adjusting Pump Settings

Adjustments to the pump should be performed systematically based on the patient's blood glucose log, food diary indicating carbohydrate intake, and the current pump settings. There are several software programs available to download information from the pump. It is worthwhile to emphasize that adjusting pump setting is an ongoing process.

12.4.1   Adjusting the Basal Rate(s)

Patients with type 2 DM should check blood glucose minimally four times a day at fasting and after each meal. Patients with type 1 DM should check at six times a day before and after each meal.

If the basal rate is correct, the patient should be able to eat late or to skip meals without having highs or lows. The basal rate can be tested overnight as described below:

1. Test blood glucose at bedtime (at least 4 h after a bolus). If blood glucose is >100 mg/dL, proceed with the test.
2. Do not eat a bedtime snack.

3. Check blood glucose at 3 am and at 7 am. If you go back to sleep after the 7 am check, repeat check on waking.
4. If blood glucose at all checks is within 30 mg/dL of the bedtime blood glucose, then the basal rate is correct.
5. If the blood glucose is more than 30 mg/dL either high or low at any check, then the basal rate should be adjusted 2–3 h prior to the rise or fall.

> How to adjust basal insulin:
> If basal rate >1 u/h, adjust 0.1–0.2.
> If basal rate 0.5–1 u/h, adjust 0.05–0.1.
> If basal rate <0.5, adjust 0.025–0.05.

12.4.2   Temporary Basal Rate

Some pumps allow a temporary basal rate to be set for up to 24 h. The temporary rate does not repeat, and it overrides the usual basal rate(s) during the time it is active. This temporary setting can be used during exercise or for other times such as long plane trips.

12.4.3   Adjust the Insulin-to-Carbohydrate Ratio (ICR)

Test the ICR as follows:

1. Test blood glucose; if blood glucose is between 70 and 140 mg/dL, proceed with the test.
2. Take calculated bolus insulin and eat a low-fat meal.
3. Test at 2 and 4 h after the meal.
4. Do not eat any additional carbohydrates during the test period.
5. Do not correct if the 2 h is high.
6. If blood glucose at 4 h is >30 mg/dL below target, increase the ICR.
7. If blood glucose at 4 h is >30 mg/dL above target, decrease the ICR.

> How to adjust the ICR: (typical adjustment is 10–20%)
> If ICR <10, adjust 1–2 points.
> If ICR 10–20, adjust 2–3 points.
> If ICR 21–30, adjust 3–5 points.
> If ICR 31–50, adjust 5–10 points.
> If ICR >50, adjust 10–20 points.

12.4.4   Adjusting the Insulin Correction Factor (ICF)

Check the accuracy of insulin correction in the following manner:

1. When BG is high, take corrective insulin.
2. Do not eat unless there are symptoms of hypoglycemia.
3. Check at 2 and 4 h.
4. If blood glucose is low at 4 h or symptoms of hypoglycemia were present, increase the ICF.
5. If blood glucose is high at 4 h, decrease the ICF.

> How to adjust the ICF:
> If ICF <30, adjust 3–5 points.
> If ICF 30–60, adjust 5–10 points.
> If ICF 61–100, adjust 10–15 points.
> If ICF >100, adjust 25 points.

12.5   Insulin Infusion Sites

The infusion site can be any area where there is a reasonable amount of subcutaneous fat. If it is possible to "pinch an inch," the site is usable. The abdomen is a common site, but other possible sites include the back of the arm, the outer thigh, the hip, and the upper buttock.

Leave a 2 inch area around the navel and any scars. Places that may experience pressure when sitting or from tight clothes should be avoided. Do not reuse areas that have lipodystrophy. During the latter stages of pregnancy, exercise caution when injecting into the abdomen over the pregnant uterus.

To avoid developing breakdown of the fat tissue (lipodystrophy), infusion sites should be rotated every 48 h ideally and every 72 h at a minimum. Change sites immediately if there is pain, sign of infection, or concern that the site is no longer usable such as persistent elevated blood glucose. Sites should be rotated in an organized manner. It is recommended to start at one side of the body and move 2 inches to identify the next site. When that part is exhausted, move to the next. As example, move across the abdomen in 2 inch increments, next move down 2 inches, and move across the abdomen in the opposite direction. Then move to the thigh and the other thigh, to the hip, and so forth. The idea is that by the time you are back to the abdomen, the previously used sites will have time to heal. There are phone apps that keep track of site rotations and provide a reminder when it is time to rotate.

12.6   Insulin Pump During Labor

Labor is physiologically similar to a prolonged period of exercise. While it is certainly possible to use the pump during labor, patients are usually focused on other things, and it is a reasonable option to allow the medical team to assess and manage blood glucose. In a study comparing women who continued pump use during labor to women on an intravenous insulin drip, no difference was found in mean and median glucose levels or episodes of hypoglycemia between groups [4]. If the pump is used during labor, monitor blood glucose hourly, and give small boluses as needed. Discontinue the pump temporarily after delivery due to the precipitous drop in insulin requirement that will occur and may last up to 24 h. Postpartum pump use can be resumed at prepregnancy settings for basal rate, boluses, and ICR and ICF.

12.7   Insulin Pump and Breastfeeding

Studies of the use of the insulin pump during breastfeeding are limited. Women who choose to use the pump while breastfeeding should be aware that breastfeeding women require 2000–2500 more calories per day.

During breastfeeding blood glucose can drop rapidly. Consider using a temporary basal rate with up 50% reduction during and for 1 h after nursing [5].

12.8   Patient Education and Training for the Insulin Pump

Patients require extensive education and training to avoid adverse events and for successful use of the device [6]. The education required for pump use falls out of the scope of this book. Topics that should be covered include [1]:

Filing the pump reservoir
Tubing
Priming the pump
Button pushing—how to give boluses
Pump alarms and error messages
Insertion of infusion sets
Infusion site infections and reactions
Changing pump settings

When a change in pump is made or the pump is upgraded, patients should be trained on the technical aspects of the new pump.

12.9   Patient Safety

The insulin pump is a complex medical device. New features are added frequently, and in order to use this device, patients must be knowledgeable [7]. Pumps can fail for a number of reasons including electrical, mechanical, software, or user error. Every patient on the pump and the family members of pump patients should be trained on the recognition and management of hypoglycemia and hyperglycemia.

12.9.1   Hyperglycemia

Uncorrected hyperglycemia can lead to diabetic ketoacidosis (DKA). Pregnant women are prone to develop DKA at a lower blood glucose level than when not pregnant.

When blood glucose >250 mg/dL occurs without a known explanation, the pump should be evaluated to insure that the infusion set is in place without leaks or crimps and that the prior bolus was delivered. Also investigate the infusion site for redness or signs of infection. A correction bolus can be given, but if it does not correct, the infusion set should be replaced and the reservoir refilled with new insulin.

Stacking is the process of delivering multiple boluses before the previous bolus has had time to work. Stacking should be avoided as it will lead to hypoglycemia that may be difficult to correct.

A backup plan should be in place to use injection therapy.

Pumps do experience mechanical failure. Pump settings should be written down, and instructions on setting the pump should be readily available.

12.9.2   Hypoglycemia

All patients should have an emergency glucagon kit. The kit should be replaced every year.

Symptoms of hypoglycemia should be evaluated by checking blood glucose.

If symptoms of hypoglycemia are present, stop all activity and check blood glucose.

If the patient can't check blood glucose, initiate treatment presumptively.

It seems obvious, but patients should be informed that if they are driving, they should pull off the road.

Use the rule of 15 to correct blood glucose <70 mg/dl:

1. Eat 15 g of rapid-acting carbohydrate (if blood glucose <50 mg/dL, start with 30 g).
2. Recheck blood glucose in 15 min.
3. If blood glucose <70 mg/dL, go back to step 1 and repeat.

After hypoglycemia has resolved, check to see that the bolus and basal settings are correct.

15 g of rapid-acting carbohydrate is:
1 tbsp of honey
1 tbsp of corn syrup
4–5 saltine crackers
3–4 glucose tablets
½ cup of unsweetened juice
8–9 jellybeans
2 tbsp sugar
½ cup of regular soda

12.9.3 Illness/Sick Days

During an illness, blood glucose may increase due to the release of stress hormones. During pregnancy, nausea and vomiting is a common complaint. Decreased food intake may cause the body to burn fat resulting in ketones. Elevated blood glucose in the presence of ketones in the urine is concerning. Diabetic ketoacidosis is a significant risk particularly in type 1 DM pregnant patients on the pump. On sick days and during periods of decreased food intake, a sick-day protocol should be followed:

1. Check blood glucose as scheduled or q4 h.
2. If blood glucose is >240 mg/dL, check urine ketones.
3. For trace ketones give a correction dose using a pen or syringe (not the pump), and increase PO intake of water or sugar-free fluids.

4. For moderate to high ketones:

- Use a pen or syringe to give a correction dose that is equivalent to 10% of the total daily dose (TDD).
- Change the infusion site and make sure that the pump is functioning correctly.
- Increase PO intake of water or sugar-free fluids.

5. Check blood glucose and ketones in 2 h.
6. If blood glucose continues to be high or moderate to large ketones, continue contact with the diabetes team, or present to the emergency room.

12.9.4   General Safety Measures

Patient should wear identification stating that they are diabetic and on the insulin pump.

Patient should have a supply of syringes in case the pump malfunctions.

Carry extra supplies for the pump.

Always carry fast-acting carbohydrates in case of hypoglycemia.

Never go to bed with a low battery on the pump.

Never ignore symptoms of hypoglycemia.

When flying, don't check supplies in baggage.

Carry a list of pump settings.

The pump can be worn through the scanner at the airport but should be removed for MRIs and X-rays.

Change the time setting on the pump when traveling to different time zones.

12.10   Summary

The insulin pump is designed to provide physiologic availability of insulin. During pregnancy, the use of the insulin pump in appropriately selected patients is associated with improved glycemic control.

References

1. Grunberger G, Abelseth JM, Bailey TS, Bode BW, Handelsman Y, Hellman R, Jovanovic L, Lane WS, Raskin P, Tamborlane WV, Rothermel C. Consensus Statement by the American Association of Clinical Endocrinologists/American College of Endocrinology insulin pump management task force. Endocr Pract. 2014;20(5):463–89. doi:10.4158/EP14145.PS.
2. Farrar D, Tuffnell DJ, West J. Continuous subcutaneous insulin infusion versus multiple daily injections of insulin for pregnant women with diabetes. Cochrane Database Syst Rev. 2007;3:CD005542. doi:10.1002/14651858.CD005542.
3. Cohen O, Keidar N, Simchen M, Weisz B, Dolitsky M, Sivan E. Macrosomia in well controlled CSII treated Type I diabetic pregnancy. Gynecol Endocrinol. 2008;24(11):611–3. doi:10.1080/09513590802531062.
4. Drever E, Tomlinson G, Bai AD, Feig DS. Insulin pump use compared with intravenous insulin during labour and delivery: the INSPIRED observational cohort study. Diabet Med. 2016;33(9):1253–9. doi:10.1111/dme.13106.
5. Riviello C, Mello G, Jovanovic LG. Breastfeeding and the basal insulin requirement in type 1 diabetic women. Endocr Pract. 2009;15(3):187–93. doi:10.4158/EP.15.3.187.
6. Jayasekara RS, Munn Z, Lockwood C. Effect of educational components and strategies associated with insulin pump therapy: a systematic review. Int J Evid Based Healthcare. 2011;9(4):346–61. doi:10.1111/j.1744-1609.2011.00228.x.
7. Rule AM, Drincic A, Galt KA. New technology, new errors: how to prime an upgrade of an insulin infusion pump. Jt Comm J Qual Patient Saf. 2007;33(3):155–62.

Chapter 13
Diabetic Ketoacidosis

Lisa E. Moore

> **Fast Facts**
>
> - Diabetic ketoacidosis (DKA) is defined by the triad of hyperglycemia, metabolic acidosis, and ketosis.
> - DKA has been identified in type 2 diabetes and in gestational diabetes though it is very rare.
> - The most common precipitants of DKA are infection and failure to take prescribed insulin.
> - DKA is a medical emergency.

13.1 Pathophysiology

The lack of insulin, either absolute as in type 1 diabetes or relative as in type 2 diabetes, causes cells to be unable to take up glucose. The body believes it is starving and releases glucagon which initiates gluconeogenesis and glycogenolysis. Metabolism of fatty acids creates ketones which can be used

L.E. Moore, MD, FACOG
Department of Obstetrics and Gynecology, Texas Tech University
Health Sciences Center El Paso, Paul L. Foster School of Medicine,
El Paso, TX, USA
e-mail: lisa.e.moore@ttuhsc.edu

© Springer International Publishing AG 2018
L.E. Moore (ed.), *Diabetes in Pregnancy*,
https://doi.org/10.1007/978-3-319-65518-5_13

by the brain as alternate energy source. As these ketones accumulate, the blood pH becomes increasingly more acidic. Absence of insulin, or resistance to insulin during pregnancy, causes glucose to remain in the blood stream instead of being taken up by cells. Gluconeogenesis and glycogenolysis also increase the amount of glucose in the blood. As the amount of glucose in the blood increases, the osmolarity of the blood increases creating an osmotic gradient in which water enters the intravascular space and is then removed by the kidneys (an osmotic diuresis). This further concentrates the glucose and ketones in the blood which pulls more fluid into the intravascular space. Severe dehydration is the result. Additionally, bicarbonate is not reabsorbed by the kidney tubules during the diuresis. The final result is diabetic keto-acidosis in which the patient has a severe volume deficit, blood glucose is elevated, the pH of the blood shows a metabolic acidosis with an anion gap, and the amount of ketones in the blood and urine is high.

13.2   How Does Pregnancy Increase the Risk of DKA?

The developing fetus requires a continuous source of glucose and amino acids. To achieve this, pregnant patients undergo physiologic adaptations such as increased insulin resistance and accelerated starvation in which gluconeogenesis and lipolysis are activated earlier during pregnancy than when not pregnant. The insulin resistance makes more glucose available for the fetus but also increases maternal serum blood glucose. Accelerated starvation with initiation of lipolysis and gluconeogenesis increases maternal blood glucose and produces ketone bodies.

Increases in minute ventilation cause a respiratory alkalosis during pregnancy. The kidneys compensate by increasing the excretion of bicarbonate (compensated respiratory alkalosis) which ultimately causes decreased ability to buffer the acidity of ketones in the blood. The decreased buffering ability is also the reason that pregnant women go into DKA at lower levels of hyperglycemia than when not pregnant.

13.3   Clinical Presentation

There are no pathognomonic clinical findings in DKA. Patients usually present with rapid respiration (Kussmaul respirations), altered mental status, vomiting, and weakness. A fruity odor on the breath has been described due to conversion of acetoacetate to acetone. Hyperventilation is believed to help raise the blood pH by removing carbon dioxide. Metabolic acidosis and ketosis causes altered mentation and may lead to coma. Patients may give a history of excessive thirst (polydipsia) and excessive urination (polyuria). There may be physical signs associated with hypovolemia including hypotension, sunken eyes, and tachycardia, and at presentation the patient may be oliguric having peed out their intravascular volume. Abdominal pain is a common complaint.

Box 13.1: Signs and Symptoms of DKA

Hyperventilation

Tachycardia

Nausea/vomiting

Abdominal pain

Altered mental status

Fruity odor on breath

Hypotension

Sunken eyes

History of polyuria becoming oliguria

13.4   Diagnosis

The diagnosis is made by high suspicion based on symptoms and physical exam and confirmed by laboratory studies. An arterial blood gas, basic metabolic panel, liver function test panel, and a complete blood count with differential should be obtained.

Serum glucose is usually >300 mg/dL. However, DKA occurs in pregnant patients at a lower level of blood glucose and has been described in pregnant patients with normal serum glucose levels.

The arterial pH is acidotic <7.3. Bicarbonate will be low usually <15 mEq/L, and the anion gap will be >12 mEq/L.

Box 13.2: Laboratory Findings in DKA

Glucose >300 mg/dL (less in pregnancy)

pH <7.3

HCO3 <15 mEq

Anion gap >12 mEq/L

BUN increased

Cr increased

K may be normal, low, or high

Na may be normal, low, or high

13.5   Common Precipitants of DKA During Pregnancy

During pregnancy, commonplace events may push susceptible patients into DKA. These events are listed in Box 13.3.

Infection causes increased production of cortisol and catecholamines which oppose the action of insulin. Infection can reduce the rate of glucose uptake by up to 50% [1].

Nausea and vomiting lead to decreased food intake resulting in activation of gluconeogenesis and lipolysis and the creation of ketone bodies. Loss of fluid and electrolytes results in dehydration.

Beta-2 agonists such as terbutaline or ritodrine which are used for tocolysis and β-2 agonists used as inhaled treatments for asthma (e.g., albuterol, salmeterol) increase insulin secretion but also increase glycogenolysis with a net effect of increasing serum glucose [2, 3].

Steroid use increases serum glucose values. Be aware also that there may be a synergistic effect between steroids and beta-2 agonists.

Noncompliance with prescribed insulin and failure of the insulin pump resulting in overwhelming hyperglycemia are a recognized cause of DKA. Dieting, failure to take insulin in an attempt to lose weight, eating disorders such as bulimia, and outright manipulative behavior have all been associated with episodes of DKA [1].

Patients with unrecognized diabetes may present in DKA during pregnancy due to the already described physiologic adaptations to pregnancy and the resultant lowered threshold for acidosis.

Box 13.3: Common Precipitants of DKA

Infection

Failure to take insulin

Nausea/vomiting

Insulin pump failure

Glucocorticoids for fetal lung maturity

B2 Agonists used for tocolysis

Unrecognized diabetes

13.6   Management

Treatment of DKA involves replacement of the fluid deficit, replacing insulin to correct hyperglycemia, and alleviation of the precipitating cause.

Most important, during pregnancy, treat the DKA first before considering delivery. While in DKA fetal assessments will not be reassuring. Correction of DKA will improve the fetal status. Pregnancy in no way alters the management of DKA; in other words, treat the patient the same as she would be treated if she were not pregnant.

Search for a precipitating event. The most important goal is to identify and treat an infection if one is present. Obtain cultures of blood and urine and a complete blood count with differential. Obtain a chest x-ray if indicated. If possible, take a thorough history including recent illnesses, all medications, and visits to the emergency room. Ask specifically about missed doses of insulin and recent episodes of hyperglycemia and changes in diet. If the patient is using an insulin pump, ask about recent problems with the pump. This information can be obtained from family members if the patient is experiencing altered mentation.

Obtain two large bore IV's. Place a bladder catheter to evaluate output. Provide supplemental oxygen and continuous monitoring of oxygen saturation. Consider admission to a medical intensive care unit. Some protocols recommend continuous fetal monitoring after 24 weeks. Fetal monitoring may not be useful if there is no intention to intervene for fetal distress until after the mother's status is improved.

An estimate of the absolute fluid deficit is 100 cm^3/kg of body weight. Keeping track of input and output, begin IV hydration with normal saline. Give 1–2 L over the first hour followed by 150–500 cm^3/h planning to replace 75% of the calculated fluid deficit over 24 h. Total replacement should be complete in 48 h. Fluid replacement dilutes the serum glucose and increases the intravascular volume which improves tissue perfusion. Improved tissue perfusion increases renal clearance of glucose.

When blood glucose is less than 250 mg/dL, the change can be made to normal saline (0.9%) and 5% dextrose (D5NS). Use ½ normal saline (0.45%) if sodium (Na) is high.

At the same time as fluid resuscitation is started, begin intravenous dosing of regular insulin. Bolus 10 units of regular insulin (or 0.1 unit/kg of actual body weight) followed by 0.1 unit/kg/h. If the blood glucose does not decrease by at least 50 mg/dL in the first hour, double the maintenance dose. Check blood glucose levels every hour. Double the maintenance dose of insulin each hour until the blood glucose falls by a minimum of 50 mg/dL in an hour. Once the blood glucose is ≤160 mg/dL, decrease the maintenance dose to 1–2 units/h.

Continue IV insulin until blood glucose has been stable for 12 h.

Resume subcutaneous insulin injections when patient is stable and tolerating oral intake.

Software-directed algorithms for managing insulin dosing in DKA are available. There is nuance to the management of blood glucose and acidosis. Admission to an ICU with management by an experienced team is preferred.

The potassium deficit can be large. Potassium levels should be monitored every 2–4 h, and replacement should be slow. The 20–40 mEq added to each liter of IV fluid should be sufficient.

The use of bicarbonate to increase pH is controversial. Some authors recommend treating patients with a pH below 7.0 or a serum bicarbonate <5 mEq/L [4].

13.7   Fetal Consequences

The exact cause of intrauterine demise associated with DKA is unclear. Glucose and ketones are known to cross the placenta very efficiently so that fetal blood glucose levels are only 15 mg/dL less than maternal levels. In lambs, maternal ketoacidosis and hyperglycemia cause lactic acidosis and hypoxia [4]. Nonstress testing in patients with DKA is always not reassuring. Variability is absent, and persistent late decelerations may be present all of which indicates that the fetus is in distress. It is theorized that this may be due to decreased uteroplacental perfusion caused by hypovolemia which may be worsened by the reflex shunting of blood away from the uterus to protect the brain.

Outcomes of fetuses exposed to DKA have been studied in a limited fashion. There may be an adverse association between exposure to ketoacids and mental development in the offspring [4–6].

13.8   Treatment of Preterm Labor

Beta-2 agonists should not be used to treat preterm labor in patients with DKA. The tocolytic of choice has in the past been magnesium. Nifedipine can be considered with awareness that hypovolemia may exacerbate hypotension. Indomethacin is a good option as long as renal function is normal. Do not give steroids for fetal lung maturity until DKA is resolved.

13.9   When to Deliver

Delivery should be undertaken only after the maternal acidosis and hyperglycemia are corrected. If the fetus survives to that point, fetal assessments usually return to reassuring status. Fetal mortality during DKA is reported as 10–36% [1, 7]. Nonetheless, adding labor induction or the stress of cesarean delivery in addition to DKA increases the risk to the mother.

13.10   Summary

DKA is a life-threatening complication of uncontrolled diabetes. Fetal mortality during an episode of DKA is high. Prompt recognition and prompt treatment are required.

Initial Workup

1. Conduct a thorough history and physical exam. Look for a precipitating cause.
2. Place two large bore IVs.

3. Place a bladder catheter and monitor input and output.
4. Order labs: CBC with diff, ABG, metabolic panel, liver function tests, urine culture, blood culture, and chest x-ray if indicated.
5. Provide supplemental oxygen. Monitor oxygen saturation.
6. +/− continuous fetal monitoring.
7. Consider transfer to ICU.

Insulin Replacement (Begin Fluid Replacement at the Same Time)

1. Bolus 10 units of regular insulin or 0.1 unit/kg of body weight.
2. Start maintenance at 0.1 unit/kg of body weight.
3. Check blood glucose and electrolytes each hour.
4. Double maintenance dose each hour until the blood glucose drops by 50 mg/dl in an hour.
5. When blood glucose ≤160 mg/dL, decrease maintenance dose to 1–2 units/h.
6. Continue IV insulin until blood glucose stable for 12 h.
7. Do not discontinue IV insulin before initiation of subcutaneous insulin therapy.

Fluid Replacement (Begin Insulin Replacement at the Same Time)

1. Estimate fluid deficit as 100 cm³/kg of body weight.
2. Start 0.9% saline at 1–2 L/h × 2 h, followed by:
3. 150–500 cm³/h of 0.9% saline—plan to replace 75% of the water deficit in 24 h.
4. When serum glucose ≤250 mg/dL, add 5% dextrose.
5. Continue IV fluids for at least 48 h.

Electrolyte Replacement

Potassium—add 20–40 mEq to each liter.
Bicarbonate—controversial
Phosphorus—no proven benefit
Magnesium—no proven benefit

References

1. de Veciana M. Diabetes ketoacidosis in pregnancy. Semin Perinatol. 2013;37(4):267–73. doi:10.1053/j.semperi.2013.04.005.
2. Philipson LH. Beta-agonists and metabolism. J Allergy Clin Immunol. 2002;110(6 Suppl):S313–7.
3. Sears MR. Adverse effects of beta-agonists. J Allergy Clin Immunol. 2002;110(6 Suppl):S322–8.
4. Parker JA, Conway DL. Diabetic ketoacidosis in pregnancy. Obstet Gynecol Clin N Am. 2007;34(3):533–43. doi:10.1016/j.ogc.2007.08.001.
5. Rizzo T, Metzger BE, Burns WJ, Burns K. Correlations between antepartum maternal metabolism and child intelligence. N Engl J Med. 1991;325(13):911–6. doi:10.1056/NEJM199109263251303.
6. Rizzo TA, Dooley SL, Metzger BE, Cho NH, Ogata ES, Silverman BL. Prenatal and perinatal influences on long-term psychomotor development in offspring of diabetic mothers. Am J Obstet Gynecol. 1995;173(6):1753–8.
7. Sibai BM, Viteri OA. Diabetic ketoacidosis in pregnancy. Obstet Gynecol. 2014;123(1):167–78. doi:10.1097/AOG.0000000000000060.

Chapter 14
Intrapartum and Postpartum Management of Diabetes

Lisa E. Moore

Fast Facts

- Increased blood glucose in the 6 h prior to delivery is associated with an increased risk of neonatal hypoglycemia.
- During labor the goal is to keep the blood glucose between 70 and 110 mg/dL.
- Oral agents have not been studied for intrapartum use.
- During the active phase of labor, insulin requirements typically decrease significantly.
- Gestational diabetics and some type 2 diabetics may not require insulin in the active phase of labor.

L.E. Moore, MD, FACOG
Department of Obstetrics and Gynecology, Texas Tech University Health Sciences Center El Paso, Paul L. Foster School of Medicine, El Paso, TX, USA
e-mail: lisa.e.moore@ttuhsc.edu

© Springer International Publishing AG 2018   137
L.E. Moore (ed.), *Diabetes in Pregnancy*,
https://doi.org/10.1007/978-3-319-65518-5_14

14.1   Introduction

Babies born to mothers with persistent hyperglycemia are at risk of hypoglycemia in the immediate neonatal period. Controlling blood glucose in the 4–6 h preceding delivery has been shown to reduce the risk [1, 2]. Both the American College of Obstetricians and Gynecologists and the American College of Endocrinologist recommend maintaining a blood glucose between 70 and 110 mg/dL [3].

During labor the requirement for insulin is dependent on the phase of labor and on the type of maternal diabetes. During the active phase of labor, insulin requirement can decrease significantly, while the requirement for glucose may be equivalent to the amount required during vigorous exercise. In general, patients with gestational diabetes controlled with diet and exercise will not require insulin or glucose supplementation during labor. Gestational diabetic patients requiring medication to achieve euglycemia and patients with type 2 Diabetes may or may not require glucose and insulin. Type 1 patients will require both insulin and glucose.

14.2   Pre-Delivery Planning

Patients being induced

- Take usual medication at bedtime.
- Eat nothing after midnight (assuming an AM induction).
- Do not take morning medication.
- On arrival check blood glucose.
- Start insulin if needed.

Patients presenting in spontaneous labor

- On arrival check blood glucose.
- Ask when last took medication and dosage.
- Start insulin if needed.

Patients with a scheduled cesarean delivery

- Take usual medication at night.
- Eat nothing after midnight (assuming AM surgery).

- On arrival check blood glucose (patient should be fasting so should be within normal limits).
- Perform cesarean section within 2 h if blood glucose is between 70 and 110 mg/dL.
- If unable to perform surgery immediately or patient in poor control, start insulin.
- Perform cesarean section after 4–6 h of blood glucose levels between 70 and 110 mg/dL to reduce the risk of neonatal hypoglycemia.

14.3   Intrapartum Management

Frequency of blood glucose monitoring

- A1 GDM — check on presentation then q4–6 h.
- A2 GDM — check on presentation then q2–4 h. If insulin required, check q h.
- T2D — check on presentation then q2–4 h. If insulin required, check q h.
- T1D — check on presentation, begin insulin and glucose infusion, and check q h.

Preparation of insulin for infusion

- 125 units of Humalog in 250 mL NS = 1 unit of insulin/2 mL.
- 50 units of regular insulin in 500 mL NS or LR = 1 unit of insulin/10 mL.
- 10 units of regular insulin in 1000 of D5NS at 100 to 125 mL/h = 1–1.25 units of insulin per hour.

Insulin during labor

- Insulin pump — patients on the pump should discontinue the pump during labor and allow the team to manage blood glucose with the insulin drip. This allows the patient to focus on the delivery without concern about managing blood glucose levels.
- A1 gestational diabetics — no insulin required in labor.
- A2 gestational diabetics — usually do not require insulin in labor particularly if have been controlled.
- Types 1 and 2 diabetics will typically require insulin.

Insulin dosing during labor
Goal—keep blood glucose between 70 and 110 mg/dL.

- If initial blood glucose >150 mg/dL, give 3 units of IV Humalog or IV regular and start insulin drip at 2 u/h.
- If initial blood glucose 125–150 mg/dL, give 2 units of IV Humalog or IV regular and start insulin drip at 1 u/h.
- If initial blood glucose 100–124 mg/dL, give 1 unit of IV Humalog or IV regular and start insulin drip at 1 u/h.
- If initial blood glucose >65 mg/dL and ≤100, start insulin drip at 1 u/h.
- If blood glucose <65 mg/dL, start insulin drip at 0.5 u/h and D5NS at 125 mL/h at the same time. Check blood glucose in 30 min.

14.4   Postpartum Management

After delivery the insulin requirement drops precipitously. Gestational diabetics will typically no longer require medication. For T1D and T2D, rather than stopping the insulin, give half the pregnancy dose or resume the prepregnancy dose. An oral agent can be considered for patients with type 2 diabetes:

- A1 gestational diabetes: Regular diet. No need to check blood glucose.
- A2 gestational diabetes: Regular diet. Check postprandial glucose. If <150 mg/dL, no need for medication.

Type 1 IDDM
Vaginal delivery

- ADA diet and ½ of total insulin dose used in pregnancy.

Cesarean delivery
Good postpartum glucose control is important for healing.

- D5NS at 125 mL/h until tolerating PO intake. Check blood glucose q4 h. Use regular insulin sliding scale to control blood glucose.
- When tolerating PO give an ADA diet and 1/2 total pregnancy insulin.

Type 2 DM

- ADA diet.
- Check 2 h postprandial glucose. If >150 mg/dL resume insulin at ½ the pregnancy dose or consider and oral agent.

Breastfeeding

- Strongly recommended—has been shown to aid in weight loss and to assist with glycemic control.
- May require more calories in diet.

Contraception

Contraception is an important aspect of the management of patients with diabetes. Diabetes alone does not represent a contraindication to contraception. Comorbidities should be considered when counseling about contraceptive choices.

- Depo-Provera
- Combined OCP
- IUD
- Implant

All Patients with GDM should be screened for diabetes at 6-week postpartum and annually.

14.5   Summary

Keeping blood glucose between 70 and 110 mg/dL for at least 6 h prior to delivery reduces the risk of neonatal hypoglycemia. Patients with gestational diabetes will often not require medication during labor. Postpartum insulin requirements are dramatically reduced in all types of diabetes.

References

1. Kline GA, Edwards A. Antepartum and intra-partum insulin management of type 1 and type 2 diabetic women: impact on clinically significant neonatal hypoglycemia. Diabetes Res Clin Pract. 2007;77(2):223–30. doi:10.1016/j.diabres.2006.10.024.

2. de Valk HW, Visser GH. Insulin during pregnancy, labour and delivery. Best Pract Res Clin Obstet Gynaecol. 2011;25(1):65–76. doi:10.1016/j.bpobgyn.2010.10.002.
3. ACOG Committee on Practice Bulletins. ACOG practice bulletin. Clinical Management Guidelines for Obstetrician-Gynecologists. Number 60, March 2005. Pregestational diabetes mellitus. Obstet Gynecol. 2005;105(3):675–85.

Chapter 15
Fetal Macrosomia

Ellen Mozurkewich

> **Fast Facts**
>
> - The ultrasound estimation of fetal weight is imprecise at best.
> - Data is limited to suggest the frequency of ultrasound evaluation to detect macrosomia.

15.1 Definitions and Adverse Outcomes

Fetal macrosomia poses significant risks to mother and fetus in both diabetic and nondiabetic pregnancies. There are different definitions of macrosomia throughout the medical literature, including >90th, 95th, or 97th percentile for gestational age and birth weight >4000 g or >4500 g [1, 2]. In general, large for gestational age refers to weight above the 90th percentile for gestational age, while macrosomia refers to fetal weight above 4000 g [3].

E. Mozurkewich, MD, MS
Obstetrics and Gynecology, University of New Mexico,
MSC 10 5580, 1 University of New Mexico, Albuquerque,
NM 87131, USA
e-mail: Emozurkewich@salud.unm.edu

© Springer International Publishing AG 2018   143
L.E. Moore (ed.), *Diabetes in Pregnancy*,
https://doi.org/10.1007/978-3-319-65518-5_15

Several studies have evaluated macrosomia in terms of birth weight sufficient to be associated with adverse pregnancy and neonatal outcomes. For example, in a recent retrospective study of the US Linked Birth-Infant Death Cohort dataset from 1995 to 2004 encompassing 30,831,694 singleton term live births and 38,053 stillbirths, Ye et al. evaluated risk for stillbirth, neonatal death, and 5-min Apgar score >4 according to birth weight subgroups [1]. As the main outcome of the study, the authors created a composite perinatal mortality and morbidity index (PMMI), which included stillbirth, neonatal death, and a 5-min Apgar score less than four. They estimated ideal birth weights according to White, Black, and Hispanic ethnic groups [1]. The analysis was predicated on the assumption that perinatal mortality would form a J-shaped distribution with mortality decreasing up to an ideal birth weight and then increasing above it [1, 4, 5].

For this study, the authors define macrosomia as birth weights that exceeded the nadir of the mortality curve and categorized infants according the following birth weight percentiles: 75th, 90th, 95th, and 97th [1]. The authors found no significant increase in these adverse perinatal outcomes until birth weight reached >97th percentile for gestational age [1]. Based on their study of birth weight relative to their composite PMMI outcome, the authors found the lowest PMMI at birth weights between 3500 and 4000 g. Above this threshold, PMMI increased. Therefore, they suggested a birth weight >4500 g in Whites and >4300 g in Blacks and Hispanics as the optimal threshold for defining macrosomia sufficient to cause increased risk for adverse perinatal outcomes [1]. The authors found that cesarean section rates increased significantly with birth weight, with an overall cesarean delivery rate of 20%. Odds ratios for adverse outcomes were greater among the vaginally delivered subgroup, but this subanalysis did not change the authors postulated cutoff points [1].

Similarly, in a Scottish cohort study encompassing 784,576 births, over the period between 1992 and 2008, birth weight above the 97th percentile was significantly associated with antepartum stillbirth with odds ratio 1.8, 95% confidence interval [CI] 1.5,2.4 [5].

Macrosomia has also been found to increase risk for intrapartum and neonatal morbidities [6–8]. A study of the US National Health Statistics database between 1995 and 1997 evaluated birth and neonatal outcomes in the 4000–4499 g group, a 4500–4999 g group, and a >5000 g group as compared to normal weight controls. The investigators found that risk for cephalopelvic disproportion, cesarean section, and birth injury was increased in a dose-dependent manner among macrosomic infants. Increasing birth weights also increased risk for birth asphyxia, meconium aspiration syndrome, hyaline membrane disease, and low Apgar score. Risk of death was only elevated in the >5000 g group as compared with normal weight controls [7].

Similarly, a retrospective cohort study including 36,241 deliveries at the University of California, San Francisco, evaluated birth outcomes stratified by the presence or absence of diabetes and the presence or absence of macrosomia (i.e., birth weight above 4000 g) [8]. The study found that macrosomia was significantly associated with RDS, hypoglycemia, shoulder dystocia, and brachial plexus injury, even in the absence of diabetes [8]. In pregnancies complicated by gestational diabetes, the risk for RDS, hypoglycemia, shoulder dystocia, and brachial plexus injury was significantly increased in macrosomic diabetic pregnancies compared to GDM pregnancies with normally growth fetuses [8].

Complications of Macrosomia

Cesarean Delivery
Birth Injury (Brachial plexus, Erbs)
Maternal pelvic floor injury
Meconium Aspiration syndrome
Low APGAR
Neonatal Hypoglycemia

15.2   Standard Versus Custom Growth Curves

Formulae for estimating fetal weight from standard biometric measurements have been constructed in a variety of different populations. All have been found to be subject to considerable imprecision [9]. Ultrasound estimation birth weights at the extremes of size have been found to be the least accurate [10]. A systematic review comparing methods of fetal weight estimation found no one method to be clearly superior to the others [10]. Similarly, a prospective observational study that evaluated methods of estimating fetal weight within 7 days of delivery found that sonographic methods of estimating fetal weight remained relatively inaccurate despite improvements in ultrasound equipment over the decade they studied (1991–2000). They found that the error in estimating fetal weights was attributable in the main to the formulae used and only to a lesser extent to inter-operator variation [9].

Some authors have suggested that the use of customized growth curves that adjust for maternal height, weight, and ethnicity may reduce misclassification errors in diagnoses of suspected macrosomia and suspected IUGR [11, 12]. A recent NICHD cohort study of longitudinal fetal growth among 2334 healthy low-risk women has documented significant differences in fetal growth according to maternal ethnicity, a finding with significant implications for classification of potentially macrosomic fetuses [13]. For example, the 95th percentile at 39 weeks was 4402 g for White women, 4226 g for Hispanic women, 4078 g for Asian women, and 4053 g for Black women [13]. However customized fetal growth curves have not yet been demonstrated to improve pregnancy or neonatal outcomes [14]. Fetal MRI is another modality that may hold promise for more accurate estimation of fetal weight at or near term [15].

15.3   Diagnosis of Macrosomia

15.3.1   Diabetic Pregnancies

There are no standard guidelines and little evidence base for frequency of ultrasound in diabetic pregnancies to screen for macrosomia. In women with pregestational diabetes, ACOG has suggested "periodic" ultrasound examinations to assess fetal growth [16]. Similarly, an ultrasound in late pregnancy to assess for macrosomia risk is suggested [16]. For women diagnosed with gestational diabetes mellitus, ACOG has recommended fetal growth assessment in the late third trimester in order to assess risk for macrosomia [17]. To our knowledge there are no studies that have ascertained the benefits or harms of this approach.

15.3.2 Nondiabetic Pregnancies

In nondiabetic pregnancies, there are no current recommendations from professional organizations regarding screening for macrosomia [14, 18], given that ACOG does not currently recommend any intervention in the instance of nondiabetic pregnancies with suspected macrosomia and estimated fetal weights below 5000 g. One factor inveighing against fetal weight estimation in nondiabetic pregnancies has been the imprecision of fetal weight estimates near term, with estimates varying from true weight by up to 20% [14].

However a recent cohort study has argued for a universal screening approach [2]. This cohort study of 3866 nulliparous women, the pregnancy outcome prediction study, compared selective, clinically indicated, ultrasound at ≥34 weeks' gestation with universal ultrasound at the same time point. This study enrolled nulliparous women with viable singleton pregnancies and did not exclude women with diabetes and other medical comorbidities. For this study, screen positive for macrosomia was defined as EFW above the 90th percentile for gestational age. The study did not include a clinical protocol for induction of labor or other interventions in the instance of pregnancies that were screen positive for macrosomia. The outcomes for this study included macrosomia >4000 g at birth, severe macrosomia >4500 g, admission to the NICU, and neonatal morbidity, defined as 5-min Apgar <7, and metabolic acidosis at birth (cord pH <7.1, and base deficit >10 mmol/L). The authors defined severe adverse neonatal outcome as live birth with neonatal death, hypoxic-ischemic encephalopathy, need for inotropes, mechanical ventilation, or severe metabolic acidosis at birth defined as cord pH <7.0 and base deficit above 12 mmol/L [2].

The authors found that when LGA fetuses with increased abdominal circumference growth velocity were identified, these fetuses were at significantly increased risk for neonatal morbidity (relative risk 2.0) and severe adverse neonatal outcome (relative risk 6.6). These relationships persisted even after adjustment for maternal diabetes. The authors concluded that universal screening for macrosomia and the use of the abdominal circumference growth velocity would identify pregnancies at risk for adverse neonatal outcomes [2].

Among the individual biometric parameters comprising the estimated fetal weight, the abdominal circumference has been demonstrated to be the most important [19]. A systematic review has compared the predictive accuracy of abdominal circumference with ultrasound EFW [19]. Diagnoses of macrosomia defined as EFW > 90th percentile, EFW > 4000 g, or EFW > 4500 g were compared with abdominal circumference >36 cm alone. The authors identified 36 studies with a total of 19,117 women. The authors constructed summary receiver operator curves and likelihood ratios for each parameter and threshold. They found macrosomia diagnosed by EFW to be equivalent to macrosomia diagnosed by AC >36 cm in the prediction of birth weight above 4000 g or above the 90th percentile for gestational age [19]. They found that positive and negative likelihood ratio for EFW in prediction of birth weight >4000 g were 5.7 (95% CI 4.3–7.6) and 0.48 (95% CI 0.38–0.60). For AC above 36 cm, the positive and negative likelihood ratios were 6.9 (95% CI 5.2, 9.0) and 0.37 (95% CI 0.30, 0.45) [19].

15.4   Causes

In diabetic women, risk for macrosomia has been related to alterations in glucose and insulin homeostasis in both early and late pregnancy. For example, Voldner et al. followed a cohort of 553 nondiabetic White women with Scandinavian heritage throughout pregnancy [20]. The investigators measured fasting glucose twice during pregnancy (14–16 weeks and 30–32 weeks) and fasting plasma insulin and HOMA-IR four times during pregnancy (14–16, 22–24, 30–32, and

36–38 weeks). The primary outcome of interest was birth weight ≥ 4200 g. This study found that among women with BMI > 27 (top quartile), the increase in fasting plasma glucose between 14 and 16 weeks and between 30 and 32 weeks was predictive of macrosomia. This relationship persisted even when pregnancies complicated by GDM were excluded. Those women in the top quartile who delivered normal weight infants did not show a significant increase in fasting plasma glucose. The investigators found that for the total cohort, fasting plasma glucose at 30–32 weeks' gestation was an independent predictor of macrosomia [20].

Similarly, a case-control study of 37 placentas from macrosomic infants and 37 normal weight infants has determined that insulin-like growth factors and their receptors are important determinants of fetal macrosomia [21]. This study compared placental insulin-like growth factor mRNA levels and their receptors. The authors demonstrated that increased placental IGF-II and IGF-IR mRNA levels were positively correlated with macrosomic birth weights [21].

15.5   Risk Factors

A number of different risk factors are associated with development of fetal macrosomia. For example, Jolly et al. evaluated 350,311 singleton pregnancies in England from 1988 to 1997 [22]. The primary outcomes for this study were birth weight above the 90th percentile for gestational age or >4000 g. Pregestational diabetes was the greatest risk factor for birth weight >90th percentile. Maternal BMI > 30 and parity >4 were the greatest risk factors for birth weight >4000 g. The most important risk factors for birth weight above the 90th percentile for gestational age were pregestational obesity (BMI) > 30 (odds ratio (OR) 2.08; confidence intervals (CI) 1.99, 2.17), pregestational diabetes (OR 6.97; CI 5.36, 8.16), gestational diabetes (OR 2.77; CI 2.51, 3.07), parity > 4 (OR 2.20; CI 2.02, 2.40), and maternal age > 40 (OR 1.22; CI 1.11, 1.35) [22].

A more recent observational study among 178,709 single pregnancies in Chinese women aimed to describe prevalence and risk factors for macrosomia and to describe associations with adverse outcomes compared with normal birth weight controls [23]. Macrosomia was defined as ≥4000 g at birth. The authors found that maternal obesity and gestational diabetes mellitus were the strongest risk factors for fetal macrosomia in this population [23].

In diabetic women, obesity and excessive weight gain during pregnancy have been associated with large for gestational age, suggesting that lifestyle modification might be important in preventing macrosomia. For example, a cohort study of Florida births over the years 2004–2008 found that prepregnancy obesity and gestational weight gain were independently associated with LGA, defined as ≥90th percentile for gestational age [24]. Similarly, a Chinese cohort study of 1049 women showed that among diabetic women, maternal BMI and pregnancy weight gain had an additive effect on birth weight [25].

A meta-analysis of 33 studies encompassing 88,599 women evaluated the effect of weight gain during pregnancies complicated by GDM on birth weight [26]. This meta-analysis found excessive pregnancy weight gain, in excess of Institute of Medicine guidelines, was associated both with macrosomia and LGA. Conversely, the study demonstrated a reduction in macrosomia among women who gained less than the currently recommended degree of weight during pregnancy [26].

Risk Factors for Macrosomia

Pregestational Diabetes
Maternal BMI > 30
Parity > 4
Excessive weight gain in pregnancy

15.6   Prevention of Macrosomia

Several trials have evaluated the effect of diet and insulin therapy on risk for macrosomia [27–29]. In the Buchanan study, subjects with GDM with abdominal circumference exceeding the 75th percentile at 29–33 weeks' gestational age were randomly assigned to diet plus insulin therapy versus diet alone. There were 30 subjects assigned to the insulin group and 29 subjects assigned to the diet alone group [27]. This small trial demonstrated that insulin therapy reduced the risk of large for gestational age infants to 13% vs 45%, $P < 0.02$ [27].

A much larger randomized trial of 1000 women who were randomly assigned to receive routine care versus diet therapy plus insulin, if needed, for gestational diabetes mellitus demonstrated that treatment of GDM significantly reduced the risk for macrosomia ≥4 kg from 21 to 10% and reduced large for gestational age, defined as birth weight above the 90th percentile, from 22 to 13% [28]. Likewise, a large multicenter trial of treatment versus usual care for among 958 women with mild gestational diabetes demonstrated that treatment reduced risk for shoulder dystocia (1.5% versus 4.0%), large for gestational age (7.1% versus 14.5%), and macrosomia (5.9% versus 14.3%) [29].

There have also been a number of trials of lifestyle interventions for gestational diabetes mellitus [30]. The Cochrane review of these trials included 15 trials that included 4501 women [30]. The lifestyle interventions that were studied included a combination of education, diet, exercise, and self-monitoring of blood glucose [30]. In six trials, that included 2994 infants, lifestyle interventions reduced risk for large for gestational age births (RR 0.60, 95% CI 0.50, 0.71). Lifestyle interventions were also found to reduce mean birth weight and macrosomia [30].

In nondiabetic women at risk, lifestyle interventions have also been proposed in order to prevent macrosomia. For example, in a randomized controlled trial including 399 non-diabetic women deemed to be at risk for GDM and for macrosomia, dietary and exercise counseling reduced the proportion of newborns who were large for gestational age from 19.7 to 12.1% ($P = 0.042$) [31]. However the intervention had no effect on the proportion of women who developed GDM [31].

Several other studies have evaluated the effect of exercise among overweight women at risk for macrosomic infants [32–34]. In a recent randomized controlled trial, Wang and colleagues randomized 300 overweight and obese pregnant women with BMI ≥ 24 to a stationary cycling exercise intervention three times weekly versus usual activity [33]. The primary outcome measure of this study was gestational diabetes mellitus. Birth weight and macrosomia were pre-specified secondary outcomes. This study demonstrated a reduction in the primary outcome of GDM diagnosis with the exercise intervention (22.0% versus 40.6%, $P < 0.001$). The investigators reported a trend toward a reduction in macrosomia >4000 g (6.3% vs 9.6%; OR, 0.624; 95% CI, 0.233, 1.673, $P = 0.3$) and diagnoses of LGA (14.3% vs 22.8%; OR, 0.564; 95% CI, 0.284, 1.121, $P = 0.1$) that did not reach significance. The study reported a 112 g reduction in mean birth weight for the exercise intervention that was statistically significant. (3345.27 g ± 397.07 g vs 3457.46 g ± 446.00 g; $P = 0.049$) [33].

A Spanish trial that included 765 nondiabetic women tested an intervention that included aerobic exercise, aerobic dance, muscular strength, and flexibility three times weekly for 50–55 min per session [34]. This study was carried out in a low-risk population and did not require obesity or overweight for entry. The primary outcome of the study was pregnancy-induced hypertension. Macrosomia was a pre-specified secondary outcome for the trial. The exercise intervention resulted in a significant reduction in macrosomia, defined as birth weight >4000 g from 4.7 to 1.8%, $P = 0.03$ [34].

However, a recent meta-analysis that evaluated nine trials including 1502 overweight and obese women did not find a reduction in macrosomia with prenatal exercise interventions. (Relative risk 0.92, 95% CI 0.72, 1.18) [32]. The reviewers did however find reductions in gestational diabetes mellitus (RR 0.61, 95% CI 0.41, 0.91) and in preterm delivery <37 weeks (RR 0.62, 95% CI 0.41, 0.95) [32].

15.7 Induction of Labor for Suspected Macrosomia in Nondiabetic Pregnancies

In the instances in which macrosomia is suspected near term, there is controversy regarding whether available inventions of induction of labor or cesarean section would improve outcomes. Some authors have postulated that induction of labor in instances of impending macrosomia might be beneficial to mother and fetus. A recent Cochrane review including four trials with 1190 non-diabetic women found that induction of labor reduced risk for shoulder dystocia (RR 0.60, 95% CI 0.37, 0.98), mean birth weight, and fractures (0.20, 95% CI 0.05, 0.79), but had no effect on the risk for cesarean section or operative vaginal deliveries [35]. This Cochrane review found no differences in other perinatal outcomes of interest; however in one included trial, induction of labor increased risk for maternal third- and fourth-degree perineal lacerations [35]. Another meta-analysis including the same four trials with 1190 participants found that induction of labor reduced the likelihood of birth weights above 4000 and 4500 g as well as fetal fractures but had no significant effect on shoulder dystocia or on mode of delivery [36].

These two meta-analyses were strongly influenced by a large European randomized controlled trial that included 822 women with estimated fetal weight above the 95th percentile for gestational age at 37–38 weeks [37, 38]. Participants were randomized to undergo induction of labor between 37 + 0 and 38 + 6 weeks' gestation versus expectant management until spontaneous onset of labor or other condition necessitating delivery. Potential participants were excluded if they had insulin-requiring diabetes; however women with diet-controlled diabetes were not excluded. The primary composite outcome of this study included shoulder dystocia, fracture of a clavicle or long bone, brachial plexus injury, intracranial hemorrhage, or death. Shoulder dystocia in this study was narrowly defined as difficulty with delivery of the shoulders that was not relieved by McRoberts maneuver or suprapubic pressure. The definition of clinically significant shoulder dystocia required 60 s or more elapsed time between the delivery of the head and the delivery of the body [37].

Significant findings in this study included a reduction of shoulder dystocia from 4 to 1%, (RR 0.47, 95% CI 0.26, 0.86); the number needed to treat was 25 [37]. Induction of labor significantly reduced the composite primary outcome (relative risk 0.32, 95% CI 0.15, 0.71). Of note, there were no brachial plexus injuries, deaths, or intracranial hemorrhages in either randomized group, although fetal fractures were non-significantly reduced by induction of labor. Induction of labor modestly increased the likelihood of spontaneous vaginal delivery completed to expectant management (RR1.14, 95% CI 1.01, 1.29) [37].

Among secondary outcomes, significant findings included increased antepartum hospital length of stay associated with induction of labor, as well as a higher proportion of infants with neonatal bilirubin concentration ≥250 mm/L in the induction of labor group. The proportion of infants requiring phototherapy after delivery was likewise increased by induction of labor (11% versus 7%, $P = 0.03$). There was no difference in neonatal intensive care unit admissions between the two groups [37].

Because of the early-term gestational age at which induction of labor was carried out in the Boulvain trial [37] and the potential increased neonatal need for phototherapy, ACOG does not currently recommend induction of labor for suspected macrosomia in nondiabetic pregnancies [6]. There is limited evidence as to whether later induction of labor at or beyond 39 weeks might reduce shoulder dystocia or improve neonatal outcomes.

15.8   Induction of Labor for Macrosomia in Diabetic Pregnancies

There is a conflicting body of evidence regarding the utility of induction of labor in diabetic pregnancies in the prevention of shoulder dystocia and macrosomia. Management has traditionally rested upon a small randomized controlled trial that included 200 women with insulin-requiring diabetes whose fetuses were judged to be appropriate for gestational age in size [39]. One hundred women per group were randomized to either induction of labor at 38 weeks' gestation or expectant management [39]. In this study, induction of labor reduced the prevalence of large for gestational age infants (23% vs 10%) and shoulder dystocia (3% vs 0%) without increasing cesarean section risk [39]. However a smaller trial involving 100 insulin-requiring women with diabetes comparing induction of labor at 38 weeks to induction of labor 40 weeks' gestation did not find any significant difference in the rate of large for gestational age infants in the 38-week induction group compared to the 40-week induction group [40].

Given the paucity of evidence from randomized controlled trials, observational studies and systematic reviews have been also used to address the question of induction of labor for macrosomia in diabetic women [41, 42]. One such cohort study reported 2604 diabetic women and compared usual care with a protocol-based approach for management of macrosomia [41]. The protocol-based approach included a policy of induction of labor for ultrasound EFW of ≥90th percentile at 37–38 weeks' gestation and elective cesarean section for EFW ≥4250 g. Compared with births among diabetic pregnancies before the protocol was instituted, the protocol reduced the shoulder dystocia rate from 2.4 to 1.1% (OR 1.9, 95% CI 1.0, 3.5). Likewise, the likelihood of macrosomia at birth (defined as ≥4000 g) was significantly reduced from 11.6 to 8.9% ($P = 0.04$). The rate of shoulder dystocia among infants delivered vaginally was 7.4% compared with 18.8% among vaginally delivered infants before institution of the labor induction protocol [41].

A 2009 systematic review that compared elective induction or cesarean section with expectant management among women with gestational diabetes evaluated evidence from one randomized controlled trial and four observational studies [2]. The authors reviewed each of the studies separately, given the heterogeneity of study designs and methods. They concluded that a policy of labor induction at term might reduce macrosomia, defined as birth weight >4000 g, as well as shoulder dystocia, but that the quality of available evidence was low and more trials are needed [42].

15.9   Mode of Delivery

There are no available randomized controlled trials to guide choice of mode of delivery for the fetus with suspected macrosomia. Thus clinical decision-making has rested upon two decision analysis studies by Rouse et al. and by Herbst [43, 44]. The Rouse study constructed a decision analysis model that compared (1) routine care without the use of ultrasound estimation of fetal weight, (2) ultrasound with elective cesarean section for EFW $\geq$4000 g, and (3) ultrasound and elective cesarean section for EFW $\geq$4500 g [43]. The main outcome measure for this study was shoulder dystocia with brachial plexus injury. Analyses were carried out separately for diabetic and nondiabetic pregnancies. The study estimated the number of additional cesarean section procedures and costs per permanent brachial plexus injury averted. The authors estimated that 3695 cesarean sections would need to be performed for nondiabetic women with ultrasound EFW $\geq$4500 g to prevent one brachial plexus injury. For diabetic pregnancies with EFW $\geq$4500 g, 443 cesarean sections would need to be performed to prevent one brachial plexus injury [43].

The Herbst study constructed a decision model comparing (1) elective cesarean section, (2) labor induction at 38–39 weeks, and (3) expectant management for nondiabetic macrosomic infants with EFW >4500 g [44]. This analysis found that expectant management was the most cost-effective strategy, yielding a cost of $4014.33 per injury-free child, compared to labor induction at $5165.08 per injury-free child or elective cesarean section at $5212.06 per injury-free child [44].

More recently a cohort study encompassed 24 years of births at the Galway University Hospital, Ireland. This study evaluated mode of delivery and neonatal outcomes of 201 births of macrosomic infants with birth weight at or above 5000 g. This study reported a 7.1% incidence of shoulder dystocia among nulliparous women who underwent labor and a 4.3% incidence of shoulder dystocia among parous women who labored [45]. Forty-four percent of the nulliparous women and 12% of the parous women in this study ultimately required intrapartum cesarean section. The overall Erb's palsy rate in the study was 1.3%. The authors concluded that a randomized controlled trial is needed to more fully evaluate the risks and benefits of elective cesarean section for suspected macrosomia [45].

15.10 Summary

Suspected fetal macrosomia remains a controversial area for clinical decision-making. Ultrasound diagnosis of macrosomia remains imprecise despite improvements in technology. There is some intriguing evidence that exercise may reduce risk for gestational diabetes and potentially macrosomia among overweight and obese women who are at risk to give birth to macrosomic infants. In the instances in which macrosomia or impending macrosomia have been diagnosed in nondiabetic women, there is considerable controversy whether the benefits of labor induction outweigh the potential harms. There is very limited evidence suggesting benefit for induction of labor in diabetic women. Recommendations for elective cesarean sections to prevent shoulder dystocia rest upon decision analytic models evaluating costs to avert brachial plexus injuries. Given the rarity of these events, as well as the medicolegal climate, it is unlikely that a definitive trial of elective cesarean section to prevent brachial plexus injury among pregnancies complicated by suspected macrosomia will ever be carried out.

References

1. Ye J. Searching for the definition of macrosomia through an outcome-based approach. PLoS One. 2014;9(6):e100192.
2. Sovio U. Universal versus selective ultrasonography to screen for large for gestational age infants and associated morbidity. Ultrasound Obstet Gynecol. 2017.
3. Araujo Júnior E, Peixoto AB, Zamarian ACP, Elito Júnior J, Tonni G. Macrosomia. Best Pract Res Clin Obstet Gynaecol. 2017;38:83–96.
4. Zhang X. How big is too big? The perinatal consequences of fetal macrosomia. Obstet Gynecol. 2008;198(5):1–6.
5. Moraitis AA. Birth weight percentile and the risk of term perinatal death. Obstet Gynecol. 2014;124(2):274–83.
6. American College of Obstetricians and Gynecologists' Committee on Practice Bulletins—Obstetrics. Practice bulletin no. 173: fetal macrosomia. Obstet Gynecol. 2016;128(5):195.
7. Boulet SL. Macrosomic births in the United States: determinants, outcomes, and proposed grades of risk. Obstet Gynecol. 2003;188(5):1372–8.
8. Esakoff TF. The association between birthweight 4000 g or greater and perinatal outcomes in patients with and without gestational diabetes mellitus. Obstet Gynecol. 2009;200(6):1–4.
9. Anderson NG. Sonographic estimation of fetal weight: comparison of bias, precision and consistency using 12 different formulae. Ultrasound Obstet Gynecol. 2007;30(2):173–9.
10. Dudley NJ. A systematic review of the ultrasound estimation of fetal weight. Ultrasound Obstet Gynecol. 2005;25(1):80–9.
11. Mongelli M. Reduction of false-positive diagnosis of fetal growth restriction by application of customized fetal growth standards. Obstet Gynecol. 1996;88(5):844–8.
12. Mikolajczyk RT, Zhang J, Betran AP, Souza JP, Mori R, Gülmezoglu AM, et al. A global reference for fetal-weight and birthweight percentiles. Lancet. 2011;377(9780):1855–61.
13. Buck Louis GM. Racial/ethnic standards for fetal growth: the NICHD fetal growth studies. Obstet Gynecol. 2015;213(4):1–449.
14. Committee on Practice Bulletins—Obstetrics and the American Institute of Ultrasound in Medicine. Practice bulletin no. 175: ultrasound in pregnancy. Obstet Gynecol. 2016;128(6):241.
15. Malin GL. Antenatal magnetic resonance imaging versus ultrasound for predicting neonatal macrosomia: a systematic review and meta-analysis. BJOG. 2016;123(1):77–88.

16. ACOG Committee on Practice Bulletins. ACOG practice bulletin. Clinical management guidelines for obstetrician-gynecologists. Number 60, march 2005. Pregestational diabetes mellitus. Obstet Gynecol. 2005;105(3):675–85.

17. Committee on Practice Bulletins-Obstetrics. Practice bulletin no. 137: gestational diabetes mellitus. Obstet Gynecol. 2013;122(2):406–16.

18. Bricker L. Routine ultrasound in late pregnancy (after 24 weeks' gestation). Cochrane Libr. 2015;29(6):CD001451.

19. Coomarasamy A. Accuracy of ultrasound biometry in the prediction of macrosomia: a systematic quantitative review. BJOG. 2005;112(11):1461–6.

20. Voldner N. Increased risk of macrosomia among overweight women with high gestational rise in fasting glucose. J Matern Fetal Neonatal Med. 2010;23(1):74–81.

21. Jiang H. Levels of insulin-like growth factors and their receptors in placenta in relation to macrosomia. Asia Pac J Clin Nutr. 2009;18(2):171–8.

22. Jolly MC. Risk factors for macrosomia and its clinical consequences: a study of 350,311 pregnancies. Eur J Obstet Gynecol Reprod Biol. 2003;111(1):9–14.

23. Wang D. Risk factors and outcomes of macrosomia in china: a multicentric survey based on birth data. J Matern Fetal Neonatal Med. 2017;30(5):623–7.

24. Kim SY. Association of maternal body mass index, excessive weight gain, and gestational diabetes mellitus with large-for-gestational-age births. Obstet Gynecol. 2014;123(4):737–44.

25. Chen Q. Associations between body mass index and maternal weight gain on the delivery of LGA infants in Chinese women with gestational diabetes mellitus. J Diabetes Complicat. 2015;29(8):1037–41.

26. Vieceli C. Weight gain adequacy and pregnancy outcomes in gestational diabetes: a meta-analysis. Obes Rev. 2017;18(5):567–80.

27. Buchanan TA. Use of fetal ultrasound to select metabolic therapy for pregnancies complicated by mild gestational diabetes. Diabetes Care. 1994;17(4):275–83.

28. Crowther CA, Hiller JE, Moss JR, McPhee AJ, Jeffries WS, Robinson JS. Effect of treatment of gestational diabetes mellitus on pregnancy outcomes. N Engl J Med. 2005;352(24):2477–86. doi:10.1056/NEJMoa042973.

29. Landon MB. A multicenter, randomized trial of treatment for mild gestational diabetes. N Engl J Med. 2009;361(14):1339–48.

30. Brown J. Lifestyle interventions for the treatment of women with gestational diabetes. Cochrane Libr. 2017;5:CD011970.
31. Luoto R. Primary prevention of gestational diabetes mellitus and large-for-gestational-age newborns by lifestyle counseling: a cluster-randomized controlled trial. PLoS Med. 2011;8(5):e1001036.
32. Magro-Malosso ER. Exercise during pregnancy and risk of preterm birth in overweight and obese women: a systematic review and meta-analysis of randomized controlled trials. Acta Obstet Gynecol Scand. 2017;96(3):263–73.
33. Wang C. A randomized clinical trial of exercise during pregnancy to prevent gestational diabetes mellitus and improve pregnancy outcome in overweight and obese pregnant women. Obstet Gynecol. 2017;216(4):340–51.
34. Barakat R. Exercise during pregnancy protects against hypertension and macrosomia: randomized clinical trial. Obstet Gynecol. 2016;214(5):1–8.
35. Boulvain M. Induction of labour at or near term for suspected fetal macrosomia. Cochrane Libr. 2016;22(5):CD000938.
36. Magro-Malosso ER. Induction of labour for suspected macrosomia at term in non-diabetic women: a systematic review and meta-analysis of randomized controlled trials. BJOG. 2017;124(3):414–21.
37. Boulvain M, Senat M, Perrotin F, Winer N, Beucher G, Subtil D, et al. Induction of labour versus expectant management for large-for-date fetuses: a randomised controlled trial. Lancet. 2015;385(9987):2600–5.
38. Norwitz ER. Induction of labour for fetal macrosomia: do we finally have an answer? BJOG. 2017;124(3):422.
39. Kjos SL. Insulin-requiring diabetes in pregnancy: a randomized trial of active induction of labor and expectant management. Obstet Gynecol. 1993;169(3):611–5.
40. Worda K. Randomized controlled trial of induction at 38 weeks versus 40 weeks gestation on maternal and infant outcomes in women with insulin-controlled gestational diabetes. Wien Klin Wochenschr. 2017. doi:10.1007/s00508-017-1172-4.
41. Conway DL. Elective delivery of infants with macrosomia in diabetic women: reduced shoulder dystocia versus increased cesarean deliveries. Obstet Gynecol. 1998;178(5):922–5.
42. Witkop CT. Active compared with expectant delivery management in women with gestational diabetes: a systematic review. Obstet Gynecol. 2009;113(1):206–17.

43. Rouse DJ. The effectiveness and costs of elective cesarean delivery for fetal macrosomia diagnosed by ultrasound. JAMA. 1996;276(18):1480–6.
44. Herbst MA. Treatment of suspected fetal macrosomia: a cost-effectiveness analysis. Obstet Gynecol. 2005;193(3):1035–9.
45. Crosby DA. Obstetric and neonatal characteristics of pregnancy and delivery for infant birthweight 5.0 kg. J Matern Fetal Neonatal Med. 2017:1–5. [Epub ahead of print].

Chapter 16
The Ultrasound Evaluation of the Diabetic Pregnancy

Carla Ann Martinez

Fast Facts

- Pregestational diabetes is associated with a two- to ninefold increased risk for a congenital anomaly or birth defect.
- Cardiovascular and central nervous system defects are the most common anomalies.
- Caudal regression is 200 times more frequent in infants of diabetic mothers than nondiabetic mothers.
- HbA1c greater than 10% is associated with a 22% risk of a congenital anomaly.

C.A. Martinez, MD
Division of Maternal Fetal Medicine, Department of Obstetrics and
Gynecology, Texas Tech University Health Sciences Center El Paso
Paul L. Foster School of Medicine, El Paso, TX, USA
e-mail: Carla.martinez@ttuhsc.edu

© Springer International Publishing AG 2018   163
L.E. Moore (ed.), *Diabetes in Pregnancy*,
https://doi.org/10.1007/978-3-319-65518-5_16

16.1   Introduction

Pregnancies complicated by pregestational diabetes (type 1 or type 2) are at increased risk for miscarriage, congenital anomalies or birth defects, fetal growth disturbances (macrosomia and intrauterine fetal growth restriction), and stillbirth. It is controversial as to whether gestational diabetes poses an increased risk for anomalies to the fetus, as these patients may reflect undiagnosed type 2 diabetics. Pregestational diabetes (PGD) increases the risk two- to ninefold higher than the baseline population risk and has been shown to correlate with maternal glycemic control, translating into an increase from 2 to 3% in the general population to 3 to 19% in the diabetic patient [1]. The poorer the maternal metabolic control is at the time of conception, the higher the risk for a birth defect. The anomalies in the fetus can vary and have been reported to affect all organ systems. The most common birth defects seen in diabetic pregnancies involve the cardiovascular, central nervous, and musculoskeletal systems, with at least 50% of anomalies affecting the cardiovascular and central nervous systems.

Maternal hyperglycemia is a known teratogen to the developing embryo. Poor maternal glycemic control during organogenesis and embryogenesis increases the risk for anomalies. Studies have consistently shown a linear relationship between maternal glycemic control and the rate of birth defects and spontaneous abortion [1–3]. The reported risk of spontaneous abortion was 12.4% with a first trimester HbA1c less than or equal to 9.3% and increased to 37.5% with a HbA1c greater than 14.4% (RR 3.0; 95% CI, 1.3–7.0) [2]. Likewise, the risk of major malformation was 3.0% with a HbA1c less than or equal to 9.3% and 40% when greater than 14.4% (RR 13; 95% CI, 4.3–40.4) (Table 16.1) [2]. Well-controlled PGD at the time of conception is associated with a reduced risk of birth defects; The recommended HbA1c threshold is < 6.5%. Earlier studies have reported no anomalies in cohorts with HbA1c less than 8.9% [3], while later studies have identified congenital anomalies in pregnancies

TABLE 16.1 Risk of malformation related maternal first trimester HbA1c

HbA1c			
SD above mean	Percentage	Percent malformations	RR (95% CI)
<6	≤9.3	3	1.0
6.1–9.0	9.4–11.0	5.2	1.7 (0.4–1.7)
9.1–12.0	11.1–12.7	4.3	1.4 (0.3–8.3)
12.1–15.0	12.8–14.4	38.9	12.8 (4.7–35.0)
>15.0	>14.4	40.0	13.2 (4.3–40.4)

$N = 303$ insulin-requiring diabetics. Adapted from Greene et al. [2]. *SD* standard deviation, *RR* relative risk

with HbA1c as low as 6.6 and 5.4% early in the pregnancy [1]. So while improved maternal glycemic control reduces the risk of congenital anomalies, it does not reduce it to the baseline population risk.

16.2   First Trimester Ultrasound

Ultrasound evaluation of the diabetic pregnancy is performed for the usual obstetric indications. Early ultrasound in the first trimester is recommended to determine viability, due to the higher rate of miscarriage, and an estimation of gestational age, which is important for delivery planning.

Early fetal anatomy evaluation at the time of the nuchal translucency screening can identify some birth defects early in pregnancy, especially in those with elevated HbA1c. Nuchal translucency (NT) screening is performed between 11.0/7 and 13.6/7 weeks. An increased NT is associated with congenital anomalies, aneuploidy, and multiple syndromes. While pregnancies complicated with PGD are not associated with an increased risk for aneuploidy, an increased NT further raises the risk for a congenital anomaly. An enlarged NT is defined as greater than or equal to 3 mm or greater than the 99th percentile for the crown rump length Fig. 16.1.

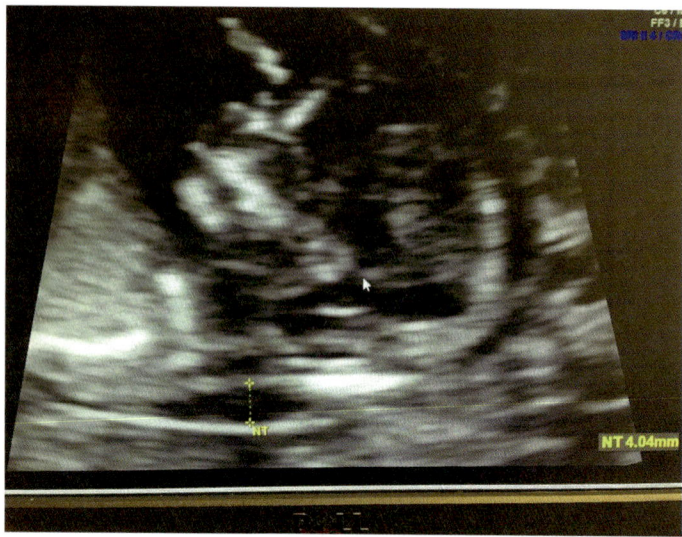

FIGURE 16.1 Enlarged nuchal translucency

Cardiac defects are the most common isolated anomalies associated with an increased NT and the most common anomalies in the general population and in pregnancies with PGD. Both are an indication for fetal echocardiography in the second trimester. In experienced centers, early evaluation of the fetal anatomy including cardiac anatomy can be achieved via transabdominal and transvaginal scanning and can identify anomalies early such as cardiac defects, anencephaly, and abdominal wall defects. The neural tube closes at day 28, poor maternal glycemic control at the time of conception will increase the risk for neural tube defects. Anencephaly in the late first trimester can be easily identified, thus allowing for safer termination of pregnancy if desired (Fig. 16.2).

16.3   Second Trimester Ultrasound

Detailed evaluation of the fetal anatomy at 18–20 weeks will identify most anomalies. Detection of fetal anomalies in the PGD can be challenging with the increasing rates of maternal

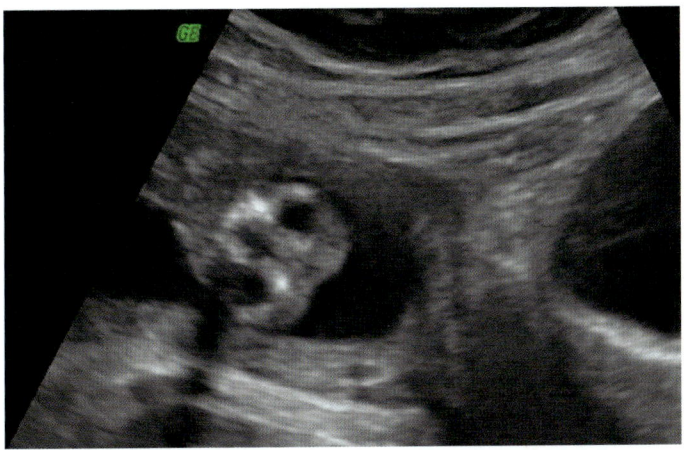

FIGURE 16.2 Anencephaly

obesity, which can limit adequate visualization of the fetus. Detailed evaluation of the fetal heart is recommended and fetal echocardiography is typically performed at 22 weeks. Numerous studies have shown a variety of congenital anomalies associated with PGD [1, 4–6]. A large population-based European database involving 18 EUROCAT registry from 1990 to 2005 demonstrated a spectrum of anomalies [4]. The most common anomalies associated with PGD were congenital heart defects (CHD) and central nervous system defects.

16.4   Screening for Congenital Heart Defects

Congenital heart defects are the most common defects seen in the general population and are increased in pregnancies complicated by PGD. In the EUROCAT cohort, isolated congenital heart defects were associated with an odds ratio (OR) of 2.07 and were the most common anomaly in the cohort, with atrial septal defects and ventricular septal defects having the highest prevalence (Figs. 16.3 and 16.4) [4, 5]. Other congenital heart defects include coarctation of the aorta and transposition of the great vessels, common

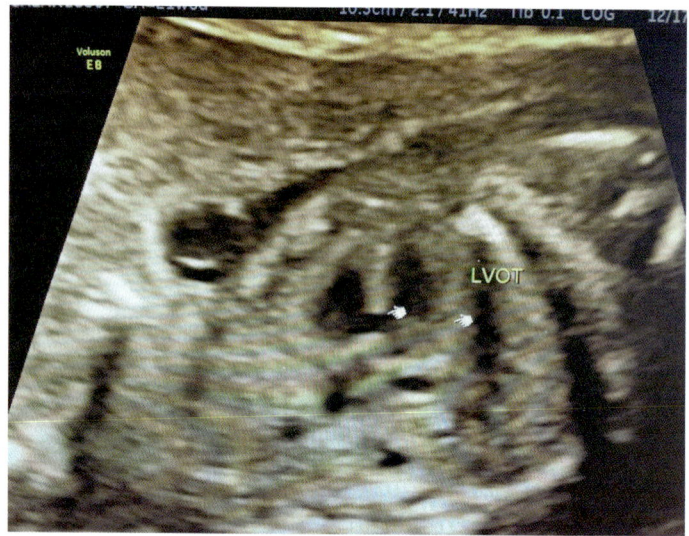

FIGURE 16.3 VSD

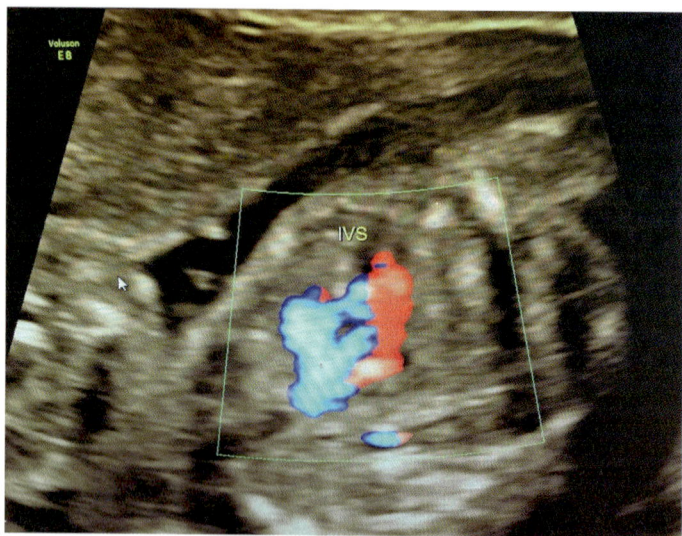

FIGURE 16.4 VSD with color Doppler

arterial truncus, single ventricle, pulmonary valve stenosis, hypoplastic left heart, and atrioventricular septal defects [4]. In a recent nationwide cohort study from Denmark, investigators examined the risk of CHDs in pregnancies exposed to PGD from 1978 to 2011 [5]. The prevalence of PGD in pregnancy in Denmark is much lower than in North America, 0.36 versus 1%. They showed a fourfold increased risk for CHD in pregnancies with PGD than pregnancies without diabetes. This trend remained constant over time. Mothers who suffered from complications from diabetes had a higher risk to have a fetus with a CHD than those who did not. The relative risk also did not differ in those treated with insulin versus oral hypoglycemics. They also observed the risk for noncardiac defects was 66% higher in patients with PDG versus without [5].

Ultrasound screening for congenital heart defects should include detailed evaluation of the fetal heart. Evaluating only the four-chamber view will miss 50% of CHD, while adding the outflow tracts will further increase the detection rate of conotruncal defects (tetralogy of Fallot, pulmonary atresia with VSD, double outlet right or left ventricle, truncus arteriosus, transposition of the great arteries). In some centers, referral for fetal echocardiography is standard practice, while in other centers it is limited to referral of those patients with an abnormal detailed evaluation or with markedly elevated HbA1c.

16.5   Screening for Neural Tube Defects

When screening for neural tube defects, one can use ultrasound alone or in combination with maternal serum alpha-fetoprotein (MSAFP). MSAFP median levels are lower in patients with PGD. With the combination of a higher risk for neural tube defects and a lower median MSAFP produced by the pregnancy, a lower threshold MSAFP value is used to have the same screen negative predictive value as in nondiabetic pregnancies. MSAFP values less than 1.5 MoM in PGD

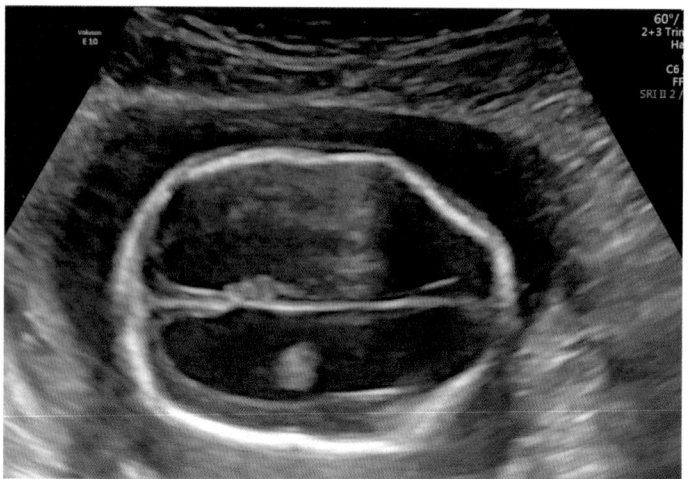

FIGURE 16.5 Lemon-shaped calvarium with bilateral ventriculo-megaly

pregnancies versus 2.5 MoM in nondiabetic pregnancies is commonly used for a screen negative result. Central nervous system defects consisting of anencephaly, encephalocele, spina bifida, and hydrocephaly have been associated with pregnancies with PGD [1, 4].

Indirect ultrasound findings associated with spinal dysraphism or spina bifida include scalloping of the front bones of the fetal cranium known as the lemon sign and ventriculomegaly (Fig. 16.5). Downward displacement of the cerebellum with herniation of the cerebellar tonsils through the foramen magnum results in the characteristic banana sign (Fig. 16.6). The sagittal view of the fetal spine shows the irregular bony spine, disruption of the fetal skin, and appearance of a cystic sac that is characteristic of a meningomyelocele. This can be seen in 2D and 3D imaging when the fetus is in the proper plane (Figs. 16.7 and 16.8). Figures 16.5–16.8 are all from the same fetus at 20 weeks.

Caudal regression syndrome or sacral agenesis is a rare congenital anomaly resulting in a spectrum of structural defects of the caudal region [7]. This can include incomplete development of the sacrum and lumbar vertebrae and can be

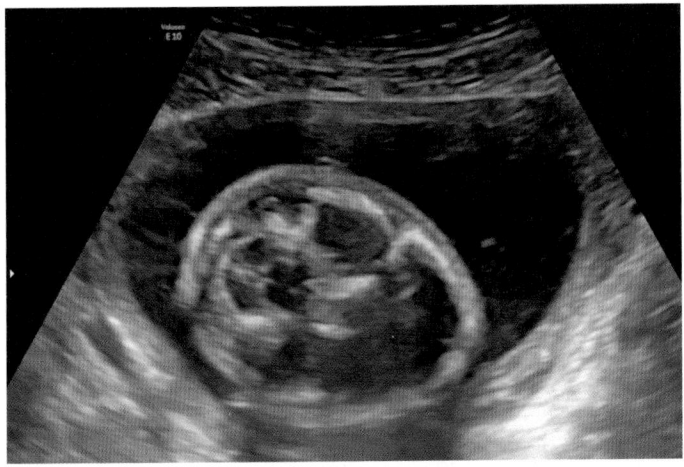

Figure 16.6 Banana sign cerebellum curved around midbrain

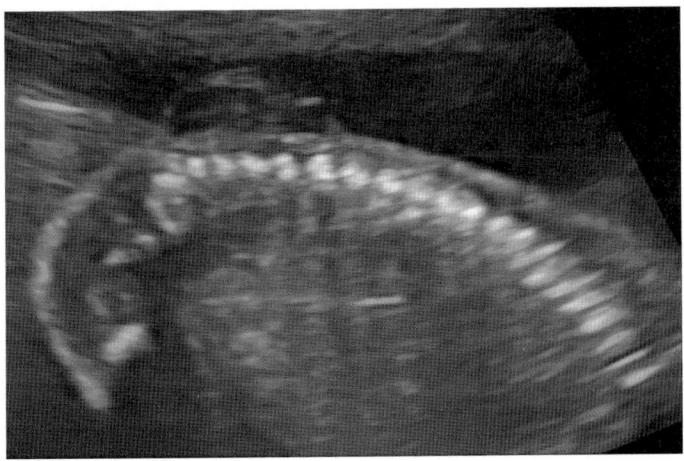

Figure 16.7 Sagittal view of the fetal spine shows the irregular bony spine, disruption of the fetal skin, and appearance of a cystic sac in 2D

associated with closed or open spinal dysraphism and varying genitourinary abnormalities including bilateral renal agenesis. It has been historically associated almost exclusively with PGD, though sporadic cases in nondiabetic patients occur. It

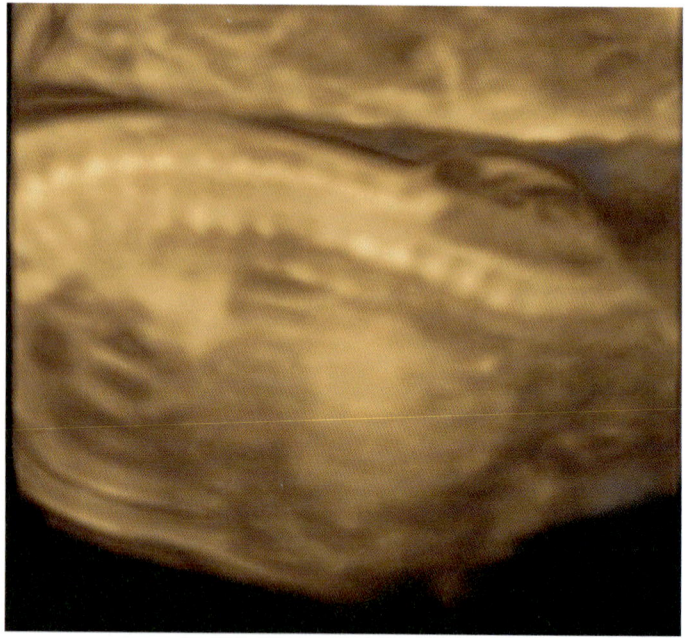

FIGURE 16.8 Same image is shown in 3D

has been reported to occur 200 times more frequently in infants of diabetic mothers than nondiabetics [1, 4, 6]. Ultrasound findings of sacral agenesis can be subtle (Figs. 16.9 and 16.10) [7]. Depending on the level of the defect the fetus may have associated lower extremity malposition known as the "tailor's posture" or "Buddha pose." More severe findings of caudal regression with open neural tube defect and renal agenesis can be challenging due to the lack of amniotic fluid. MRI can help confirm the diagnosis if needed (Fig. 16.11).

Associated genitourinary abnormalities that can be seen in PGD pregnancies include bilateral renal agenesis, hydronephrosis, and multicystic dysplastic kidney. In bilateral renal agenesis, the lack of amniotic fluid can make the diagnosis challenging. The characteristic ultrasound finding of absent kidneys in the renal fossa results in the adrenal glands

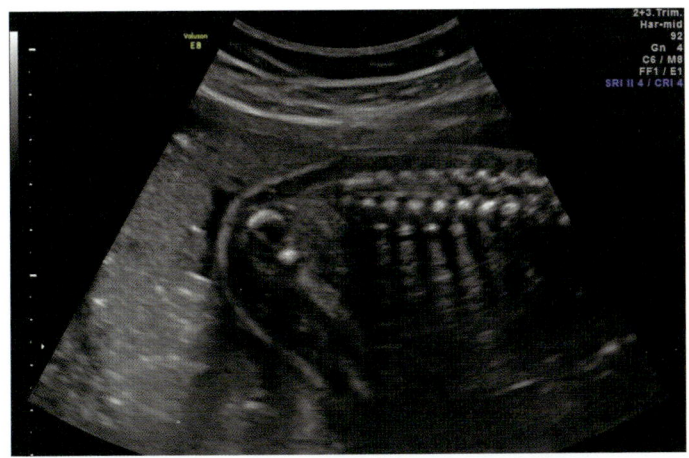

FIGURE 16.9 Sacral agenesis 2D

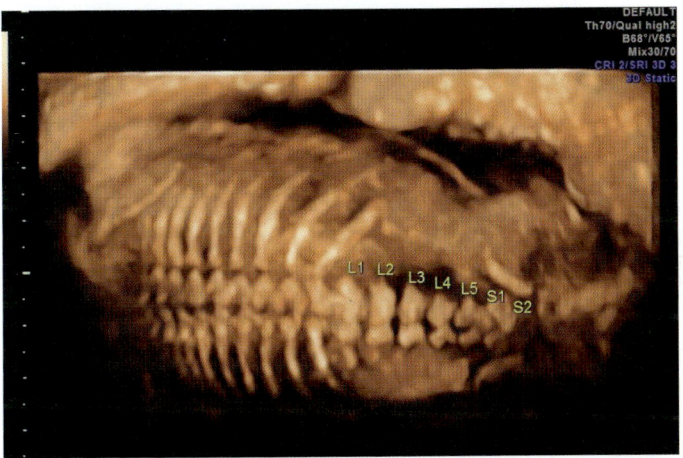

FIGURE 16.10 Sacral agenesis 3D

being more prominent. The prominent adrenal glands then fill the renal fossa, and this is known as the lying down adrenal sign (Fig. 16.12). Color Doppler evaluation of the abdominal aorta will lack visualization of the bilateral renal arteries (Fig. 16.13).

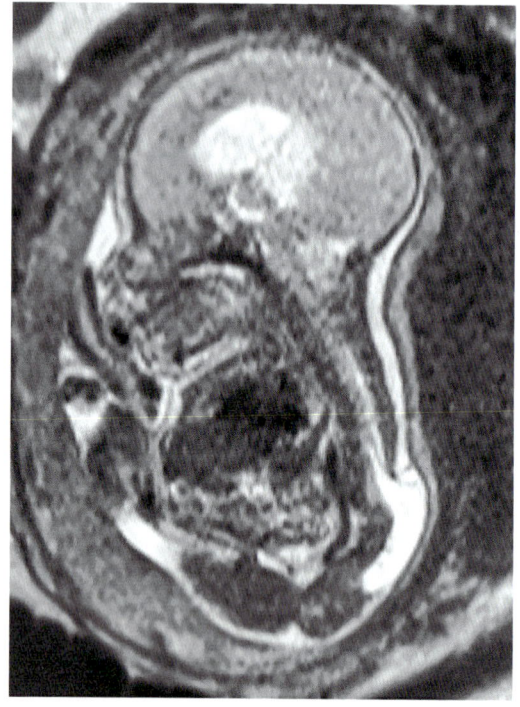

FIGURE 16.11 MRI demonstrating caudal regression syndrome with bilateral renal agenesis

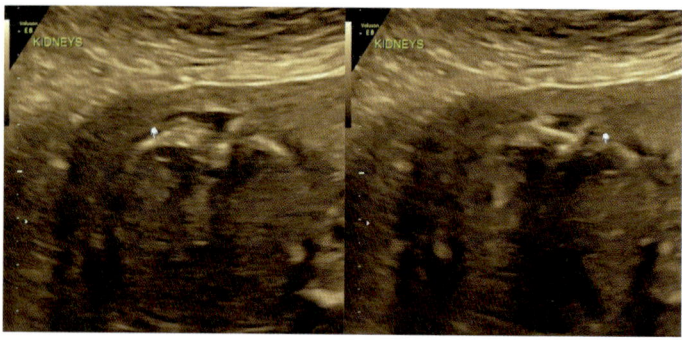

FIGURE 16.12 Bilateral renal agenesis, prominent adrenals "laying down sign"

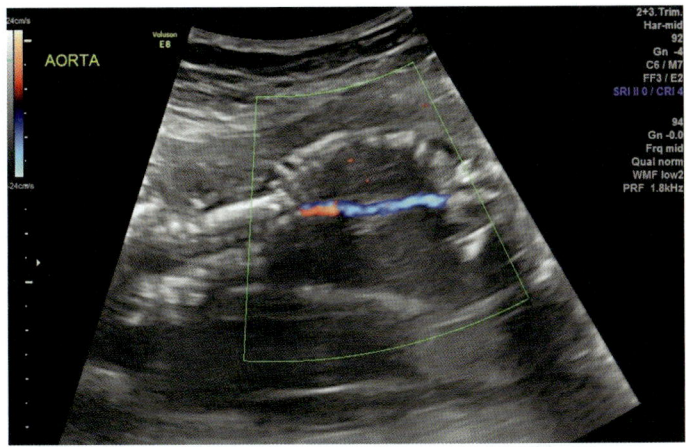

FIGURE 16.13 Bilateral renal agenesis with anhydramnios. Note the lack of renal arteries coming off the abdominal aorta

16.6   Follow-Up Ultrasounds Assessing Fetal Growth

Macrosomia occurs in 42–62% of pregnancies complicated by type 1 diabetes, in 30–56% of those with type 2 diabetes, and in 10–20% with gestational diabetes [10]. Fetal macrosomia as defined by the American College of Obstetricians and Gynecologists (ACOG) implies growth beyond an absolute birth weight, typically defined as 4000–4500 g, regardless of the gestational age, while large for gestational age implies a birth weight equal to or greater than the 90th percentile for a given gestational age. There is no universally accepted definition for macrosomia, and given the associated maternal morbidity and neonatal risks associated with larger birth weights, ACOG has recommended a continuum be used (Box 1) [8].

Box 1 Risks Associated With Increasing Birth Weight

Birth weight of 4000–4499 g with increased risk of labor abnormalities and newborn complications

Birth weight of 4500–4999 g with additional risk of maternal and newborn morbidity

Birth weight of 5000 g or greater with additional risk of stillbirth and neonatal mortality

Due to alterations in fetal growth in pregnancies with PGD both accelerated, increasing the risk for macrosomia, and impaired growth, increasing the risk for intrauterine fetal growth restriction (IUGR), assessment of the fetal growth is recommended. Fetal morbidity and mortality are associated with both macrosomia and IUGR. There are no large trials to determine when the optimal timing of fetal growth assessment should occur. Most authorities recommend assessment in the late second trimester and early third trimester (e.g., 26–28 weeks) when accelerated fetal growth typically becomes apparent and repeated at 3–4 week intervals in the third trimester to monitor fetal growth. In general patients with high insulin resistance and/or requirements are more prone to have macrosomic fetuses, while those with maternal vasculopathies are at risk for impaired fetal growth. However, this should be tailored to the patient's glycemic control, physical exam, and assessment of the fetal growth. Poor glycemic control may warrant earlier ultrasounds and prompt evaluation of fetal well-being.

Neonatal birth weight is predictive of neonatal morbidity. Estimation of fetal weight near the time of delivery is often used for delivery planning. Unfortunately, ultrasound assessment of fetal macrosomia has not shown to be precise. In a retrospective clinic study looking at the accuracy of 36 commonly used weight estimation regression formulas in evaluating macrosomic fetuses greater than 4000 g, none attained a detection rate and false positive rate for fetuses greater than or equal to 4500 that could be used for clinical recommendation. One of the most commonly used formulas,

Hadlock IV, had the highest detection rate for fetuses with a birth weight greater than 4500 g (74.5%) but has a false positive rate of 31.5% [9].

Macrosomic infants of diabetic mothers tend to have increased fat mass and a higher body fat percentage, and their growth profiles have been shown to be disproportionate. Head circumference (HC) to abdominal circumference (AC) ratios have been evaluated as markers of accelerated fetal growth. Ultrasound evaluation of both macrosomic and non-macrosomic fetuses of type 1, type 2, and gestational diabetics versus controls has shown to have a smaller AC early in pregnancy and larger AC at term. The HC/AC ratio at term is lower in all diabetic subgroups except in non-macrosomic type 2 diabetic cases [10].

Impaired fetal growth is a risk factor for PGD with pre-existing vasculopathies or coexisting chronic hypertension. IUGR is defined as the estimated fetal weight below the 10th percentile. Once IUGR is identified, the fetal well-being should be monitored via Doppler velocimetry to monitor the uteroplacental resistance via fetal arterial and venous vessels. Increased placental resistance will result in increases in umbilical artery impedance with diminished, then absent, and then reversed end diastolic flow (Fig. 16.14). Fetal activity should also be assessed with biophysical profiles done at weekly intervals in conjunction with Doppler velocimetry of the umbilical artery. Serial growth ultrasounds are performed every 3 weeks to monitor the fetal growth. The rationale is to identify those fetuses at highest risk for in utero demise and may require preterm delivery.

16.7   Polyhydramnios

Polyhydramnios is a known complication of pregnancies complicated by PGD. It is defined as a total amniotic fluid index of greater than 25 cm or a deepest vertical pocket of 8 cm (Fig. 16.15). The reported prevalence is 1.5–66% of pregnancies with PGD. There are several proposed mechanisms for this, and the most commonly accepted

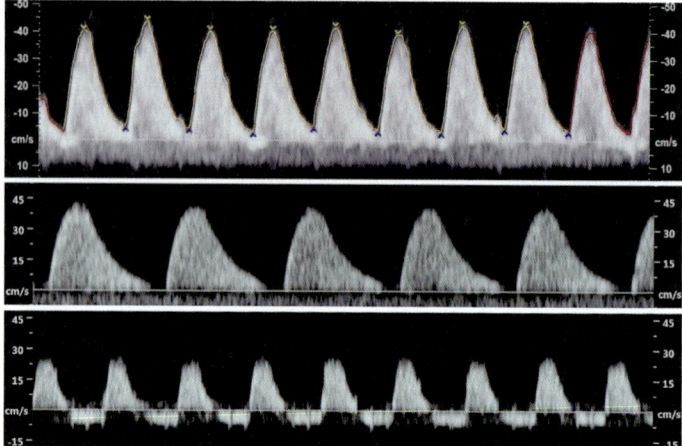

FIGURE 16.14 Umbilical artery Doppler velocimetry progressing from elevated in the *top panel*, to absent end diastolic flow in the *middle panel* to reversed end diastolic flow in the *bottom panel*. The mother had type 2 diabetes with chronic hypertension and end-stage renal disease on dialysis

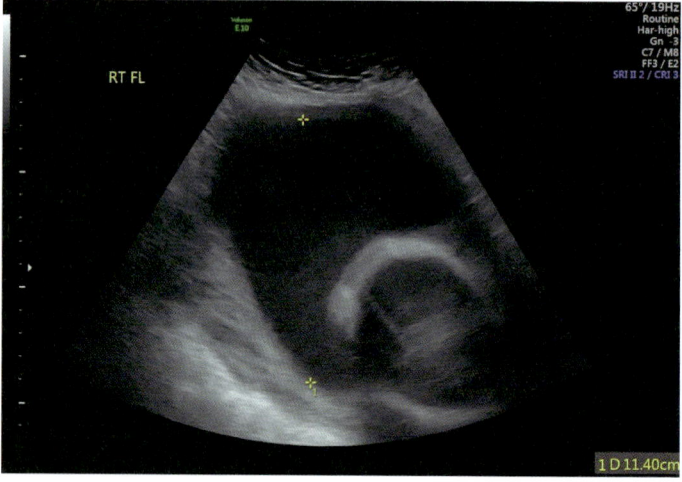

FIGURE 16.15 Polyhydramnios demonstrated by deepest vertical pocket

theory is it thought to be due to fetal polyuria secondary to fetal hyperglycemia as a result of maternal hyperglycemia. It is associated with poor maternal glycemic control when not due to a fetal congenital anomaly such as esophageal atresia. It has not been associated with poor fetal outcomes but increases the risk of iatrogenic preterm delivery [11].

16.8 Assessment of Fetal Well-Being

Intrauterine fetal demise (IUFD) occurs less frequently today with better glycemic control but is higher than the general population. The mechanism for fetal demise is thought to be related to the increased oxygen demands of the fetus due maternal hyperglycemic that results in fetal hyperglycemia and hyperinsulinemia. If these demands are not met, the fetus will become acidotic and is at risk for demise. Maternal vasculopathies can also increase this risk resulting in impaired placental perfusion and fetal growth restriction.

ACOG recommends fetal surveillance in pregnancies complicated by PGD [12]. Fetal activity monitoring by fetal kick counting, nonstress testing (NST), biophysical profiles (BPP), or contractions stress tests are all available methods. Formal fetal testing is recommended to be initiated at 32–34 weeks gestation. This should be tailored to maternal glycemic control as those patients with poor control may warrant fetal testing earlier. The frequency and method of fetal testing is up to the provider as no one method has been shown to be superior. If NST is chosen, it is recommended to perform twice weekly NST, due to the increased risk for stillbirth with only weekly testing of 1.9/1000 [13]. The BPP evaluates the acute and chronic well-being of the fetus by examining the NST and ultrasound examination of fetal breathing, fetal movement, fetal tone, and amniotic fluid index. Two points are given for each component with a total score of 10/10. The NST can be eliminated if all the ultrasound components of the BPP are met with no change in the validity of the test. The rate of stillbirth within 1 week with a BPP score of 8/10 or 10/10 is 0.8/1000 [13]. A modified BPP which consists of ultrasound evaluation of the AFI combined with a NST is also used. It has the same stillbirth rate as a complete BPP within 1 week of a normal test of 0.8/1000 [13].

16.9   Summary

Ultrasound is a key component in caring for pregnancies complicated by pregestational diabetes due to the increased risk of congenital anomalies and fetal growth disturbances and in the assessment of fetal well-being. Detailed evaluation of the fetus is recommended as cardiovascular, and central nervous system defects are the most common anomalies. Due to the high rates of macrosomia and associated neonatal morbidities, monitoring the fetal growth is recommended.

References

1. Gabbay-Benviz R, Reece EA, Wang F, Yang P. Birth defects in pregestational diabetes: defect range, glycemic threshold and pathogenesis. World J Diabetes. 2015;6(3):481–8.
2. Greene MF, Hare JW, Cloherty JP, et al. First-trimester hemoglobin A1 and risk for major malformation and spontaneous abortion in diabetic pregnancy. Teratology. 1989;39:225–31.
3. Lucas MJ, Leveno KJ, Williams ML, et al. Early pregnancy glycosylated hemoglobin, severity of diabetes and fetal malformations. Am J Obstet Gynecol. 1989;161:426–31.
4. Garne E, Loane M, Dolk H, et al. Spectrum of congenital anomalies in pregnancies with pregestational diabetes. Birth Defects Res A Clin Mol Teratol. 2012;94(3):134–40.
5. Øyen N, Diaz LJ, Leirqul E, et al. Prepregnancy diabetes and offspring risk of congenital heart disease: a nationwide cohort study. Circulation. 2016;133(23):2243–53.
6. Mills JL. Malformations in infants of diabetic mother. Teratology. 1982;25(3):385.
7. Kumar Y, Gupta N, Hooda K, et al. Caudal regression syndrome: a case series of a rare congenital anomaly. Pol J Radiol. 2017;82:188–92.

8. ACOG Committee on Practice Bulletins. Fetal macrosomia. Practice bulletin No. 173. American College of Obstetricians and Gynecologists. Obstet Gynecol. 2016;128:e195–209.

9. Hoopman M, Abele H, Wagner N, et al. Performance of 36 different weight estimation formulae in fetuses with macrosomia. Fetal Diag Ther. 2010;27:204–13.

10. Hammoud NM, Visser GHA, Peters SAE, et al. Fetal growth profiles of macrosomic and non-macrosomic infants of women with pregestational or gestational diabetes. Ultrasound Obstet Gyneol. 2013;41:390–7.

11. Idris N, Wong SF, Thomae M, et al. Influence of polyhydramnios on perinatal outcome in pregestational diabetic pregnancies. Ultrasound Obstet Gynecol. 2010;36:338–43.

12. ACOG Committee on Practice Bulletins. Pregestational diabetes mellitus. Practice bulletin No. 60. American College of Obstetricians and Gynecologists. Obstet Gynecol. 2005;105:675–85.

13. ACOG Committee on Practice Bulletins. Antepartum fetal surveillance. Practice bulletin No. 145. American College of Obstetricians and Gynecologists. Obstet Gynecol. 2014;124:182–92.

Chapter 17
Antepartum Testing

Valerie Rappaport

> **Fast Facts**
>
> - Causes of fetal loss in diabetic pregnancy are multifactorial.
> - No method of antenatal surveillance has proven superior.

17.1   Introduction

Over the past 30 years, antepartum fetal surveillance strategies have become a routine part of management of diabetic pregnancy. This testing is initiated in the third trimester to identify pregnancies at imminent risk of stillbirth and allow early delivery. Equally important, antepartum testing identifies those pregnancies with a low risk of in utero demise thus allowing safe continuation of the pregnancy thereby avoiding prematurity associated neonatal morbidity and mortality.

V. Rappaport, MD
Division of Maternal Fetal Medicine, Department of Obstetrics and Gynecology, University of New Mexico Health Sciences Center, Albuquerque, NM 87131, USA
e-mail: vrappaport@salud.unm.edu

© Springer International Publishing AG 2018
L.E. Moore (ed.), *Diabetes in Pregnancy*,
https://doi.org/10.1007/978-3-319-65518-5_17

17.2   Historical Outcomes of Diabetic Pregnancy

Historically, diabetes complicating pregnancy was considered to confer such a grave prognosis for the mother that no focus was placed on pregnancy management for the purpose of fetal survival. In the pre-insulin era, maternal mortality associated with pregnancy was over 50% with fetal mortality exceeding 65%. In the classic textbook, *Williams Obstetrics*, 1st edition, published in 1903, the complete discussion of management of the diabetic pregnancy was given in the following passage: "In patients suffering from diabetes, gestation sometimes exerts a very deleterious influence upon the course of the disease. Accordingly, if the patient's condition becomes alarming, labour should be induced" [1]. The discovery of insulin in 1922 and its use in diabetic pregnancy management led to a dramatic improvement in maternal mortality and morbidity. However, in 1933 a review of diabetic pregnancy outcomes concluded that, although maternal mortality was decreased in the post-insulin age, there had been little improvement in fetal and neonatal outcomes and survival with the most important cause of fetal loss being poor control of the maternal disease with ketoacidosis and fetal death [2]. By the 1940s, Dr. Pricilla White had pioneered the concept of intensive management of diabetes in pregnancy coupled with timed early delivery to improve perinatal outcomes. In 1949, she reported on her series of 439 patients which preexisting diabetes managed at the Joslin Clinic in Boston. In contrast to earlier reports, there were no maternal deaths during pregnancy. However, the perinatal loss rate after 27 weeks, while improved, was still 180/1000 births. In this group, 43% of the losses were due to third trimester stillbirth, while the remaining 56% were neonatal deaths related to birth trauma, macrosomia, and prematurity. The risk of fetal demise increased with duration of maternal diabetes and was most marked in women with vascular complications of diabetes such as retinopathy and nephropathy. In this hallmark paper, she introduced the concept of planned preterm or early term deliveries in pregestational diabetes in relation to the severity of maternal diabetes. She proposed the "White's Classification" for diabetes in pregnancy which guided classification and management of diabetes in pregnancy for many decades [3]. Integral with this concept was the recognition that long-standing diabetes, particularly in association with maternal vasculopathy, increased the risk of placental insufficiency and chronic fetal hypoxemia resulting in third trimester fetal loss. The hope was that implementation of intensive insulin treatment and strict control of maternal blood glucose levels would resolve the problem of third trimester stillbirth alleviating the need for early delivery and prematurity risks. However, this did not turn out to be true. In a review of diabetic management in 1959, Dr. White noted that late stillbirth remained a significant issue and suggested, "Early timing of the delivery remains an important part of management. It is directed against intra-uterine deaths due to vascular insufficiency in any pregnancy. Although poorly judged timing and errors in dates may turn intra-uterine into neonatal deaths, early timed deliveries have lowered viable mortality rates" [4].

The White classification was used for many years to guide successful management of pregestational diabetes as well as the addition of gestational diabetes in later years. However, fetal loss remained high. Improvements in prenatal care starting in the 1970s, which importantly included the implementation of fetal surveillance techniques, coupled with ultrasound assessment and advanced neonatal care resulted in a marked decrease in the rate of fetal death in women with pregestational diabetes. In 1960, the stillbirth rate was 150/1000 births [5]. By the 1990s, a large study from US National Center for Health Statistics analyzing over 10 million births between 1995 and 1997 reported a risk of stillbirth of 5.9/1000 in the diabetic population, including both pregestational and gestational diabetics, as compared to 4.0/1000 in the nondiabetic population [6]. This was a marked improvement; however, women with diabetes continue to experience increased risk of stillbirth, particularly at or near term. In a recent review from the United States looking at both preconception and gestational diabetes, the full-term (>36 weeks) stillbirth rate among women with diabetes was 3/1000 births, which was more than twice as high as the rate in the overall obstetric population of 1.3/1000 births [7]. For the group of women with pregestational diabetes, type 1 and type 2, the stillbirth rate continues to be higher with an estimated fivefold relative risk over baseline in on average over a number of studies [5, 8, 9].

17.3   Pathophysiology of Stillbirth

The causes of increased fetal loss in diabetic pregnancy are multifactorial. As with nondiabetic pregnancies, about half of stillbirths are associated with obstetrical events such as cord occlusion, intrauterine infection, placental abruption, and congenital malformations which may not be amenable to prevention with fetal surveillance. In addition, diabetes often coexists with other medical conditions such as obesity, hypertension, and autoimmune disease which may carry their own risks. However, insights into the pathophysiology of stillbirth in diabetes suggested that many diabetic-related fetal losses result from the common endpoint of chronic fetal hypoxia, a condition which may be detectable by antepartum pregnancy screening.

Several pathways are felt to contribute to fetal hypoxia in diabetic pregnancies. Patients with pregestational diabetes, particularly long-standing disease, have an increased risk of diabetic vasculopathy. Decreased uterine perfusion in patients with microvascular disease can lead to restricted trophoblast invasion in early pregnancy, uteroplacental blood flow, and decreased spiral artery remodeling resulting in third trimester fetal growth restriction [5]. Fetal growth restriction due to reduced uteroplacental perfusion is associated with a significant increase in the risk of stillbirth, as much as 3.4–6.5-fold over baseline. In a recent study of unexplained stillbirth, growth restriction represented the strongest risk for stillbirth after 34 weeks [10].

Acute maternal ketoacidosis a rare cause of stillbirth in developed countries and is associated with a high rate of fetal death. However, chronic unexpected fetal acidosis may also contribute to unexplained fetal death. Bradley et al. in 1991 obtained fetal blood samples by cordocentesis between 20 and 40 weeks gestation in type 1 diabetic women. He found that some fetuses in the third trimester were significantly acidotic despite lack of overt maternal ketoacidosis [11].

Another pathway to fetal hypoxia is chronic maternal hyperglycemia. This concept, known as the Pedersen hypothesis, states that maternal hyperglycemia results in fetal hyperglycemia causing fetal hyperinsulinemia [12]. High fetal insulin levels in turn drive accelerated fetal growth, and disproportionate fetal oxygen demand resulting in chronic fetal hypoxia and placental hypoxia [13]. Datta et al. reported that infusion of glucose into normal and diabetic women in labor can result in neonatal hypoxia and fetal metabolic acidosis [14]. Fetal response to chronic hypoxia results in pronounced extramedullary hematopoiesis driven by erythropoietin. Erythropoietin (EPO) is noted to be increased in amniotic fluid and plasma of poorly controlled diabetic pregnancies. Markedly increased amniotic fluid EPO levels have been described prior to stillbirth in diabetic women [15, 16]. In addition, maternal glycosylated hemoglobin (HbA1c) in the third trimester correlates directly with umbilical venous EPO at delivery, suggesting that antepartum maternal hyperglycemia is a significant factor driving chronic fetal hypoxia [17]. In a Danish review of stillbirths in type 1 diabetic pregnancy during 1990–2000, 50% of otherwise unexplained stillbirths were characterized by suboptimal glycemic control in late pregnancy [18].

Recent studies also suggest that hypoxemia-related fetal cardiac dysfunction might contribute to stillbirths in pregnancies complicated by diabetes. Elevated levels of pro B-type natriuretic peptide (pro-BNP) and Troponin T are also found in offspring of women with type 1 diabetes mellitus who had poor glycemic control during early pregnancy [19]. In the fetus, BNP functions as a vasodilator in the placental circulation and has protective autocrine effects. Troponin T is a marker of acute myocardial damage. Elevated levels BNP and troponin have been found to precede fetal death. Postmortem reports of stillborn infants of diabetic women showed these infants have heavier hearts and thicker ventricular walls [20]. These studies support the hypothesis that fetal hypoxemia failure due to cardiac dysfunction may also contribute to stillbirth in diabetic patients.

17.4   Timing of Stillbirths

Since fetal hypoxemia is felt to precede fetal death in many cases of diabetic-related fetal loss, antepartum screening strategies directed at biophysical markers of chronic fetal hypoxia presents an opportunity to monitor pregnancies at risk and plan delivery prior to irreversible fetal damage. However, limited in utero fetal therapy exists to correct chronic hypoxemia. Therefore, effective intervention is contingent on detecting fetal compromise at a gestational age where delivery would have a reasonable possibility of neonatal viability. Although some cases of diabetic fetal loss from hypoxemia occur prior to viability, most studies of diabetic stillbirth indicate the largest proportion of losses occur in the third trimester well within the range of fetal viability. Reddy et al. reported a retrospective cohort study of prepregnancy risk factors comparing 712 singleton antepartum stillbirths to 174,097 singleton live births at or after 23 weeks gestational age. The average GA for stillbirth at delivery was 31.9 weeks vs 38 5/7 for live birth. In the subset of pregnancies delivering after 36 weeks, the overall stillbirth rate was 0.8/1000; however, in women with preexisting diabetes, the term stillbirth rate was over three times higher at 3.1/1000 [9]. In a review of 84,295 births, Huang et al. found that two thirds of unexplained fetal deaths occurred after 35 weeks [21]. Therefore, the ability to detect fetal compromise though antepartum screening in the third trimester would be expected to be an effective strategy preventing fetal loss in the diabetic pregnancy.

17.5   Biochemical Screening

Initial screening in diabetic pregnancy, to prevent stillbirth, focused on biochemical markers of placental failure. Serial estriol measurements were used to assess placental function. This was later combined with fetal biophysical assessment by nonstress testing or contraction stress test. In 1985, Mashini et al. reported on combining estriol with CST testing to manage diabetic pregnancies [22]. In his series, 4% of GDM and 10% of insulin-dependent diabetics experienced a drop in estriol levels requiring early delivery. Perinatal mortality in this study was 5.6/1000 for GDM and 13/1000 for insulin-requiring diabetes which represented an improvement over the existing baseline. However, estriol measurements were cumbersome to perform, of limited availability, and ultimately were not proven to be more effective that biophysical testing. Therefore, biochemical screening has been replaced by fetal biophysical surveillance. However, there is a renewed interest in biochemical markers of fetal hypoxia and placental hypoxia. EPO has been proposed as a marker of fetal hypoxemia. Exponential increases in amniotic fluid EPO levels in high-risk pregnancies have been documented in association with fetal hypoxia [16, 23]. Other hypoxia-induced angiogenic factors such as the adipokine leptin are currently being explored [24]. Improved understanding of the biochemistry of placental function and markers of placental dysfunction may lead to new biomarkers to use for fetal surveillance.

17.6   Biophysical Screening

The predominant antenatal testing strategy used today looks at fetal physiologic responses to hypoxemia and acidosis. Control of the fetal heart rate, fetal activity levels, and muscle tone is determined by a balance of sympathetic and parasympathetic stimulation. This balance is mediated through neurotransmitters, including catecholamines and therefore can reflect physiologic responses of the fetus to stress including hypoxemia or acidosis. Fetal activity levels and muscle tone are also correlated with fetal oxygenation and have found to be altered in states of fetal hypoxia and acidosis. In prolonged hypoxemia, redistribution of fetal blood flow leads to decreased renal perfusion, fetal oliguria, and oligohydramnios. Given that fetal hypoxemia is felt to be a common pathway leading to stillbirth, surveillance for these physiologic fetal adaptations provides the ability to intervene—generally with delivery of the fetus—before progressive metabolic acidosis leads to fetal death.

Several important limitations should be kept in mind regarding antepartum biophysical testing. Fetal biophysical surveillance is an indirect measure of fetal hypoxia or acidosis. Validation studies using direct umbilical cord sampling have shown a lower mean pH in fetuses with abnormal testing indicating that this testing does correlate with fetal hypoxia with loss of fetal motion occurring at the lowest pH levels [25]. However, factors such as fetal sleep-wake cycles, neuromuscular disorders, fetal renal dysfunction, medication exposures, and prematurity may also influence biophysical testing. In the diabetic pregnancy, maternal hyperglycemia and ketoacidosis will influence fetal biophysical testing. Correction of the maternal metabolic abnormality will often resolve the fetal biophysical abnormality without requiring delivery of the fetus.

17.7   Antenatal Testing Methods

Several different approaches are currently in use clinically to assess fetal well-being and placental function.

17.7.1   Fetal Kick Counts

Maternal fetal movement monitoring is frequently recommended as a general screen for fetal health in the third trimester. This is an easy and convenient way to evaluate fetal well-being and is commonly used as universal fetal surveillance in low-risk pregnancies. There is no preferred methodology for fetal kick counts that has proven to be superior. Most commonly, patients are asked to record fetal motion once a day. A count of 10 movements in 2 hours is felt to be reassuring [26]. If decreased activity is noted, further evaluation with fetal nonstress testing or biophysical profile is recommended. Used in this way the false-positive rate resulting in iatrogenic fetal intervention is very low.

Fetal kick counting has not been specifically validated in diabetic pregnancies but is widely used as a universally accessible and patient-centered screening in the third trimester. While observational studies suggest movement monitoring can be helpful, some clinical trials in high-risk women are inconclusive [27]. For uncomplicated, diet-controlled gestational diabetics, some have suggested that fetal kick counts may be adequate for fetal surveillance due to low risk of fetal hypoxemia and the lack of studies indicating a clear benefit from other forms of fetal testing prior to term.

17.7.2   Contraction Stress Testing (CST)

The contraction stress test (CST) is based on the response of the fetal heart rate to transient decreases in fetal oxygenation with uterine contractions and is felt to be an assessment of placental reserve. Currently, the CST is not commonly used as the primary screening tool because administering the test is more invasive, cumbersome, and time-consuming than alternative screening techniques. In addition, CST results in a larger proportion of equivocal or uninterpretable test results than other testing strategies.

To perform the test, the patient is placed in the lateral recumbent position. The FHR and uterine contractions are simultaneously recorded with an external fetal monitor. An adequate uterine contraction pattern is present when there are at least three contractions lasting at least 40 seconds within a 10-min period. Contractions can be spontaneous or induced with either nipple stimulation or intravenous oxytocin. The CST is interpreted according to the presence or absence of late FHR decelerations with a positive testing showing late deceleration for 50% of contractions over a 30-minute time period or after three consecutive contractions. Relative contraindications to the CST generally include conditions that also are contraindications to labor or vaginal delivery [28].

A contraction stress test has a negative predictive value of greater than 99%, and, when used serially for antepartum surveillance, the fetal death rate is low. Observed fetal death rates are 1 to 2 per 1000 within a week of a negative test. A positive CST is predictive of fetal hypoxia or adverse outcome 70% of the time [29]. Currently, the CST is most commonly used as a backup test for a nonreactive NST and can be safely used for this purpose even in preterm gestations [30].

17.7.3   Nonstress Testing (NST)

The NST, or cardiotocometry, is one of the most common forms of antepartum surveillance and has been widely used in diabetic pregnancy over the past 4 decades. It is based on the concept that in a healthy term infant, the fetal heart rate will accelerate temporarily with fetal motion, a response that is regulated through the fetal autonomic system. If the autonomic system is depressed due to the hypoxemia or acidosis, this response will not occur [30].

To perform the NST, the patient is positioned in a semi-Fowlers or lateral recumbent position. The fetal heart rate (FHR) is monitored with an external transducer and a second external tocometer is placed to measure uterine contraction activity. A tracing of at least 20 min is obtained; however, a more extended tracing of 40 min or more may be necessary if the fetus is in a sleep state. FHR accelerations are transient peaks that reach at least 15 bpm above baseline with the total acceleration lasting 15 seconds. Nonstress testing involves monitoring the fetal heart rate for 20–60 min and is considered reactive if there are two or more accelerations during a 20-min period. It is not necessary for the FHR acceleration to remain at 15 bpms above baseline the entire

15 seconds [31]. Vibroacoustic stimulation (VAS) is often used to stimulate the fetus and reduce the time needed for a reactive test. Importantly, the use of VAS has been shown to reduce the incidence of nonreactive tests by as much as 40% [32, 33]. A reactive NST is highly predictive of fetal well-being within the subsequent days. However, a nonreactive NST has a 50–70% false-positive rate for fetal hypoxemia or placental insufficiency. Therefore, confirmatory testing is recommended prior to altering obstetrical management [31].

Fetal heart rate reactivity is influenced by fetal developmental maturity. From 24 to 28 weeks gestation up to 50% of normal fetuses and 5% of fetuses at 28–32 weeks have NSTs not reaching the 15 bpm criteria. A lower threshold for reactivity of 10 bpm lasting 10 s is commonly used to assess the fetus between 24 and 32 weeks gestational age and has been clinically validated in this age group [34].

NST is performed either once or twice a week as a screen of fetal well-being. In the diabetic pregnancy, early studies indicated a persistently elevated stillbirth rate with weekly testing with reports of fetal loss within 72 h of a reactive NST [35, 36]. This has led to widespread adoption of twice weekly testing in the diabetic pregnancy.

17.7.4   Biophysical Profile (BPP)

The BPP was introduced in the 1980s as an enhancement to NST testing which could assess both acute and chronic fetal hypoxia [30]. It is composed of five parameters. Each of the components is assigned a score of either 2 (present) or 0 (absent) depending on the following criteria:

1. Nonstress test—reactive for gestational age
2. Fetal breathing movements—one or more episodes of rhythmic fetal breathing movements of 30 s or more within 30 min
3. Fetal movement—three or more discrete body or limb movements within 30 min

4. Fetal tone—one or more episodes of extension of a fetal extremity with return to flexion, or opening or closing of a hand
5. Determination of the amniotic fluid volume—a single deepest vertical pocket greater than 2 cm

A composite score of 8 or 10 is considered normal, a score of 6 is considered equivocal, and a score of 4 or less is abnormal. Regardless of the overall score, oligohydramnios, defined as an amniotic fluid volume of 2 cm or less in the single deepest vertical pocket, as well as significant variables or decelerations on the NST should trigger further evaluation [37, 31].

Several modifications of the original BPP are commonly used in practice. In some cases, the NST can be safely omitted if other testing is normal, resulting in a normal score of 8/8 [38]. Omission of the NST in biophysical profile surveillance of the diabetic pregnancy has not been specifically validated. In some cases, other elements of the BPP cannot be interpreted with confidence in the diabetic patient as noted below, and the NST should not be omitted in these cases.

The most common modification of the BPP, referred to as the modified BPP, involves the use of the NST in combination with amniotic fluid volume. The NST is used as an early indicator of fetal hypoxia while the amniotic fluid volume is an assessment of chronic uteroplacental dysfunction. The results of the modified BPP are considered normal if the NST is reactive, and the amniotic fluid volume is greater than 2 cm in the deepest vertical pocket. The modified biophysical profile has been validated in comparison to full biophysical profile in high-risk pregnancy however not specifically in diabetics [39, 40]. When used as a primary screen for the diabetic patient, the NST portion of the modified BPP is generally performed twice weekly with once or twice weekly fluid assessment due the concern for increased stillbirth risk with weekly testing in the setting of diabetes as noted above.

While the biophysical profile is commonly used for fetal surveillance in diabetic pregnancies, there are some special considerations in the setting of maternal diabetes which may influence results. Acute maternal hyperglycemia has been found to increase fetal respiratory movements, whereas sustained maternal hyperglycemia of over 120 may result in decreased fetal motions [41, 42]. Therefore, biophysical profile should be interpreted with caution during maternal glucose instability. Polyhydramnios is a special concern in diabetes. The amniotic fluid volume is commonly increased in women with gestational diabetes. Some studies, but not all, have shown that polyhydramnios is a marker for increased stillbirth risk and adverse birth outcome [43, 44]. Due to this concern, increased amniotic fluid levels on BPP testing (maximum vertical pocket of 8 cm or AFI over 25) should be interpreted with caution in the diabetic pregnancy. Direct correlation of fetal blood pH with BPP scoring also raises concerns about the accuracy of this scoring in the diabetic pregnancy. Salvesen et al. performed cordocentesis after BPP and fetal heart rate monitoring in 41 diabetic pregnancies between 27 and 39 weeks' gestation. While there was a significant association between low BPP score and low fetal pH, the authors found that 50% of the acidemic fetuses normal BPP scores. This leads the authors to conclude that the BPP was a poor predictor of fetal acidemia in diabetic pregnancies [45].

Despite these concerns, BPP has been widely used in diabetic pregnancies and is generally felt to be a useful guide for delivery decisions resulting in improved outcomes. Although no large randomized trials exist for BPP testing in diabetes, many observational studies suggest that the BPP and modified BPP are effective tools for antepartum surveillance. Johnson et al. used the BPP as primary surveillance in a group of 50 patients with insulin-dependent diabetes, who had twice weekly testing and 188 patients with gestational diabetes, who underwent weekly testing. There were no stillbirths in this small group, and the incidence of an abnormal test was 3.3% [46]. Kjos et al. described obstetric outcomes in 2134 diabetic pregnancies including both gestational and pregestational diabetes. Using twice weekly modified BPP they found that no stillbirths occurred within 4 days of the last antepartum testing. With this testing scheme, these investigators had an exceptionally low stillbirth rate of 1.4/1000 [47].

17.8   Fetal Doppler

Recently, Doppler velocimetry has been added to the ante-partum screening strategy for diabetic pregnancies. Doppler ultrasound enables the real-time assessment in placental and fetal circulation and has been used widely in high-risk pregnancies. Studies have found a direct correlation between abnormal umbilical Doppler velocity waveforms, abnormal placental pathology, fetal hypoxemia and acidemia, and increased fetal mortality and morbidity [48]. In the well-perfused fetus with normal placental circulation, the umbilical circulation represents a low-resistance state. In disorders of placental perfusion, particularly growth restriction and hypertensive disorders, increased placental vascular resistance leads to decreased umbilical artery diastolic flow. In severe cases, diastolic flow is absent or even reversed which is associated with a significant increase in perinatal mortality. Commonly measured flow indices express the relationship between peak-systolic velocity and end-diastolic velocity as a frequency shift ratio (D) or as the mean peak frequency shift over the cardiac cycle (A). Commonly reported measures include systolic to diastolic ratio (S/D), resistance index (S-D/S), and pulsatility index (S-D/A). The technique of obtaining the Doppler trace is critical to obtaining interpretable results. To maximize interpretability, multiple waveforms should be assessed in the absence of fetal breathing, wall-filter settings should be set low enough to avoid masking low level diastolic flow, and care should be taken to avoid interference from umbilical venous flow which can be mistakenly interpreted as diastolic flow.

Umbilical artery Doppler velocimetry has not been shown to be useful as a screening tool in the low risk, well-grown fetus; however, it has been shown to be a valuable addition to standard antepartum testing in the growth-restricted fetus or pregnancies complicated by hypertensive disorder or other risk factors for placental insufficiency. A recent Cochrane review indicated the use of Doppler ultrasound in high-risk pregnancies reduces the risk of perinatal deaths and results in less obstetric interventions [49]. Doppler studies of other fetal blood vessels, including the middle cerebral artery, aortic isthmus, and ductus venosus, have been used in some studies to further define fetal risk; however, it is unclear at this time how to apply these measures to improve neonatal outcomes [50]. There are also no large studies to define appropriate timing for fetal Doppler studies; however, they are typically repeated once or twice weekly in conjunction with BPP or NST testing.

There has been conflicting data regarding the use of Doppler studies as a general screen in patients with diabetes mellitus. Some studies propose a beneficial effect, while others did not find this. In a comparison of NST, biophysical profile, and umbilical artery Doppler velocimetry, Bracero et al. found that Doppler studies were more effective than NST or BPP in identifying a subgroup of diabetic pregnancies with adverse perinatal outcome [51]. However, the incidence of stillbirth was too rare in this small study to compare the rates of stillbirth. Bracero et al. also reported Doppler screening in a series of 227 patients with diabetes and concluded that an elevated umbilical S/D ratio in combination with abnormal glycosylated hemoglobin was associated with adverse pregnancy outcome [52]. This study did not control for other risk factors associated with increased Dopplers such as intrauterine growth restriction. Wong et al. examined 104 pregnancies with preexisting diabetes with serial Doppler measurements. He found that Doppler studies had a sensitivity of 35%, specificity of 94%, positive predictive value of 80%, and negative predictive value of 68%. Only 30% of women in this study with adverse outcomes actually had abnormal Doppler studies suggesting limited use of a general screen [53]. A retrospective study of 146 patients with gestational diabetes also noted that Doppler added little clinical value unless the pregnancy was complicated by preeclampsia or intrauterine growth restriction. Reece and colleagues found that elevations of the umbilical artery systolic/diastolic ratio were significantly associated with maternal vasculopathy, hypertension and renal insufficiency, as well as intrauterine growth restriction and neonatal metabolic complications. However, they also noted elevated Dopplers in the setting of normal outcomes with well-controlled gestational diabetes [54]. The current evidence in general does not seem to support Doppler as a primary screening tool for routine fetal surveillance in the diabetic pregnancy, especially in patients with well-controlled gestational diabetes. However, Doppler does appear to be valuable in diabetic pregnancies complicated by fetal growth disorders, vasculopathy, and hypertensive disorder [49].

Fetal growth abnormalities are important predictors of adverse perinatal outcomes in diabetic pregnancies. Accelerated fetal growth is typical in gestational diabetes due to maternal hyperglycemia; however, diabetic pregnancy can also be associated with fetal growth retraction especially in long-standing pregestational diabetes or when there are other vascular complications such as hypertension. Maternal hyperglycemia may result in overstimulation of fetal growth, and maternal vasculopathy may results in growth deficiency-decreased nutrient trance and subsequent IUGR. It has been proposed that the coexistence of maternal hyperglycemia and diabetic vascular disease produces an unfavorable intrauterine environment which may falsely "normalize" the assessment of fetal growth [55]. Due to this, it is reasonable to include assessment of Doppler velocimetry in any patient with pregestational diabetes or borderline fetal growth even in the absence of overgrowth restriction, overt vasculopathy, or hypertension. Data to support this comes from a study of pregnancies complicated by type 1 diabetes, where umbilical artery Doppler velocimetry was found to be superior to NST and BPP in identifying fetuses at risk of adverse outcomes even in the absence of overt underlying vasculopathy or IUGR [51].

17.9   Efficacy of Antepartum Fetal Surveillance

Pregnant women who have diabetes appear to have improved outcomes with some form of antepartum surveillance; however, the best methods, the best timing interval for testing, the optimal gestational age to begin testing, and the more accurate interpretations of the testing are not known. There are no prospective randomized studies with sufficient power to assess these various measures. In addition, since antepartum testing has been routinely used in diabetic pregnancy for over 3 decades, the relative contribution of antepartum testing to the remarkable improvement in perinatal outcomes in diabetic pregnancies is unclear. However, in studies of high-risk pregnancy, not restricted to diabetes, normal antepartum fetal test indicates a very low risk of stillbirth within a week of testing and has led to improved outcomes. In one analysis, not restricted to diabetic pregnancy, the rate of intrauterine fetal demise following normal testing was 1.9/1000 in 5861 NSTs, 0.3/1000 in 12,656 CSTs, 0.8/1000 in 44,828 BPPs, and 0.8/1000 in 54,617 modified BPPs. Based on these data, the negative predictive value is 99.8% for the NST and is greater than 99.9% for the CST, BPP, and modified BPP [31]. The low false-negative rate of these tests is contingent on the clinical response to abnormal testing including confirmatory testing to prevent iatrogenic prematurity as well as delivery when appropriate to prevent stillbirth.

Population-based observational studies also suggest that antepartum testing and appropriate clinical follow-up can improve perinatal outcome. In one survey of stillbirth from the UK, the authors reviewed 76,356 delivered and 195 stillbirths. They noted the frequent association of IUGR with unexplained stillbirth. The overall stillbirth rate was 4.2/1000, which was a composite of a rate of 2.4/1000 in pregnancies without fetal growth restriction and 16.7/1000 in pregnancies with fetal growth restriction. Of pregnancies with fetal growth restriction, the stillbirth rate for antenatally detected cases was 9.7/1000, while the rate increased to 19.8/1000 when the IUGR was not detected during the pregnancy. The authors also noted that pregnancies with fetal growth restriction detected antenatally were delivered on average 10 days earlier than those not detected antenatally which suggested that targeted monitoring and prenatal intervention was effect in preventing fetal demise. Based on the prevalence of undetected fetal growth restriction (9.2%) and the lower risk of stillbirth when it is detected (adjusted relative risk 3.4), the authors estimated that 18.2% of stillbirths in this cohort could have been avoided through improved antenatal detection targeted care [10].

17.10   Clinical Management Protocols

There are no large randomized trials which compare the various antepartum fetal surveillance techniques, timing of testing, onset and duration of testing, the use in various subsets of diabetic patients, or interaction with early timed delivery strategies in diabetic pregnancies. Population-level observational studies commonly combine outcomes of pregestational diabetes with gestational diabetes although it has been well documented that the risk of maternal vasculopathy and in utero fetal loss are very different in these two populations. Since gestational diabetes is far more common than pregestational diabetes, these combined data may not appropriately address risk and benefits for pregestational diabetics. In addition, with current screening and aggressive management of gestational diabetes, some have argued the perinatal loss rate does not differ from baseline for the uncomplicated, diet-controlled gestational diabetic [56].

Despite these limitations in data, there is a consensus from most authorities and professional associations that antepartum fetal surveillance is an essential part of the comprehensive prenatal care for all pregnancy diabetics. There is a lack of consensus on specific testing protocols; however, some common recommendations are as follows:

Common testing protocols involve either BPP, modified BPP, or alternating NST, BPP twice weekly starting at 32–34 weeks for all pregestational diabetics, medication control gestational diabetics, and gestational diabetics with other comorbidities such as obesity or hypertension. Doppler velocimetry is recommended in addition to biophysical testing for patients with vascular complications, hypertensive disorders, and poor fetal growth.

Given the lack of definitive guidance, each center should establish a protocol based on available resources, current evidence, and patient population characteristics and apply this protocol consistently for all diabetic pregnancies.

Antepartum fetal surveillance is of unclear benefit in patients with diet-controlled, uncomplicated gestational diabetes. Available data suggest that third trimester antepartum fetal loss is not increased over baseline in this narrowly defined group. This has led to the suggestion that antepartum surveillance may be safely deferred until 40 weeks in this group [56].

Abnormal testing results should be responded to clinically however do not necessarily require immediate delivery of the pregnancy. In the diabetic pregnancy, abnormal fetal testing should always prompt an evaluation of maternal metabolic status. Fetal testing will often improve with resolution of the maternal condition.

Given the high false-positive rates of all antepartum fetal surveillance, abnormal test results are usually followed by another backup testing unless delivery is clearly indicated based on fetal condition or gestational age. Each clinical practice should establish specific guidelines within their group for follow-up of abnormal testing and apply these consistently.

Decreased fetal motion or kick counts should be evaluated by NST, BPP, modified BPP, or CST. Abnormal results from an NST or from a modified BPP generally should be followed by additional testing with either a CST or a BPP.

A BPP score of 8–10 is considered normal; however, low amniotic fluid does require independent follow-up. In addition, significant decelerations or variables on a NST tracing require further evaluation regardless of overall BPP scoring. An equivocal BPP score, 6/10, should prompt further evaluation and consideration of delivery if the GA is 37 weeks or greater. In a preterm fetus, depending on clinical circumstances, repeat testing within 24 h may be appropriate prior to making the decision to delivery. A BPP score of 4 is almost always indicates that delivery is warranted, although in some cases extended monitoring with inpatient care may be appropriate [31].

While there are no definitive randomized clinical trials to guide the timing of delivery of the growth-restricted diabetic fetus based on umbilical artery Doppler velocimetry, current society guidelines generally suggest delivery at 32 weeks or earlier if there is reversed end-diastolic flow and delivery at 34 weeks with absent end-diastolic flow. If the Dopplers show an elevated S/D or RI (>95%) but diastolic flow is still present, delivery should be considered at or beyond 37 0/7 weeks of gestation [50, 57]. As previously noted, each practice should develop a follow-up protocol-based clinical resource, patient population, and best available guidelines and follow this protocol consistently.

Normal fetal antepartum surveillance does not override other recommendations regarding timing of delivery in diabetic pregnancy. There is no evidence that antenatal surveillance without timed delivery in alignment with current guidelines results in improved perinatal outcomes [7].

17.11   Summary

1. Antepartum fetal surveillance in diabetic pregnancy is felt to improve fetal outcomes and decrease late pregnancy fetal loss in combination with meticulous glucose control and early timed delivery.

2. Serial fetal surveillance is recommended for all pregnancies complicated by diabetes. Since the best methods, timing interval for testing, the optimal gestational age to begin testing, and optimal testing follow-up strategy are unclear, each practice should establish their own protocol based on available study outcome data, available resources, professional society recommendations, and patient population.

This protocol should be consistently applied to all diabetic patients in the practice.

3. Commonly used testing strategies involve twice weekly assessment with modified BPP or biophysical profile testing starting at 32–34 weeks and continuing until delivery. In some cases of diet-controlled, uncomplicated gestational diabetes, it is reasonable to initiate antepartum testing at 40 weeks.

4. Abnormal testing raises consideration of delivery depending on the clinical situation however in general should be confirmed with backup testing especially in the case of NST or modified BPP. All abnormal testing in diabetic patients should trigger maternal metabolic assessment prior to proceeding with delivery.

5. Addition of umbilical Doppler velocimetry improves outcomes in pregnancies complicated by fetal growth restriction and hypertensive disorder and should be considered where there are concerns for diabetic vasculopathy, long-standing diabetes, fetal growth disorders, or maternal hypertension.

References

1. Williams JW. Obstetrics. New York: D. Appleton; 1903.
2. Skipper E. Diabetes mellitus and pregnancy. A clinical and analytical study (with special observations upon thirty-three cases). Q J Med. 1933;2:353–80.
3. White P. Pregnancy complicating diabetes. Am J Med. 1949;7:609–16.
4. White P. Pregnancy and diabetes, the annual review. Diabetes. 1958;7(6):494–5.
5. Dudley DJ. Diabetic-associated stillbirth: incidence, pathophysiology, and prevention. Clin Perinatol. 2007;34(4):611–26.
6. Mondestrin MA. Birth weight and fetal death in the United States: the effect of maternal diabetes during pregnancy. Am J Obstet Gynecol. 2002;187:922.
7. Little SE, Zera CA. A multi-state analysis of early-term delivery trends and the association with term stillbirth. Obstet Gynecol. 2015;126(6):1138–45.

8. Starikov R, Dudley D. Stillbirth in the pregnancy complicated by diabetes. Curr Diab Rep. 2015;15(3):11.

9. Reddy UM, Laughon SK. Prepregnancy risk factors for antepartum stillbirth in the United States. Obstet Gynecol. 2010;116(5):1119–26.

10. Gardosi J, Madurasinghe V. Maternal and fetal risk factors for stillbirth: population based study. BMJ. 2013;346(1):f108–82.

11. Bradley RJ, Brudenell JM. Fetal acidosis and hyperlacticaemia diagnosed by cordocentesis in pregnancies. Diabet Med. 1991;8(5):464–8.

12. Pedersen J. The pregnant diabetic and her newborn: problems and management. Chicago: Williams & Wilkins; 1967.

13. Philipps AF, Porte PJ. Effects of chronic fetal hyperglycemia upon oxygen consumption in the ovine uterus and conceptus. J Clin Invest. 1984;74:279–86.

14. Datta SA. Acid-base status in diabetic mothers and their infants following general or spinal anesthesia for cesarean section. Anesthesiology. 1977;3:272–6.

15. Buescher U, Hertwig K. Erythropoietin in amniotic fluid as a marker of chronic fetal hypoxia. Int J Gynaecol Obstet. 1998;60:257–63.

16. Teramo K, Kari MA. High amniotic fluid erythropoietin levels are associated with an increased frequency of fetal and neonatal morbidity in type 1 diabetic pregnancies. Diabetologia. 2004;47:1695–703.

17. Widness JA, Teramo KA. Direct relationship of antepartum glucose control and fetal erythropoietin in human type 1 (insulin-dependent) diabetic pregnancy. Diabetologia. 1990;33:378–83.

18. Lauenborg J, Mathiesen E. Audit on stillbirths in women with pregestational type 1 diabetes. Diabetes Care. 2003;26:1385–9.

19. Halse KG, Lindegaard ML. Increased plasma pro-B-type natriuretic peptide in infants of women with type 1 diabetes. Clin Chem. 2005;5:2296–302.

20. Teramo KA. Obstetric problems in diabetic pregnancy—the role of fetal hypoxia. Best Pract Res Clin Endocrinol Metab. 2010;24(4):663–71.

21. Huang DY, Usher RH. Determinants of unexplained antepartum fetal deaths. Obstet Gynecol. 2000;95(2):215–21.

22. Mashini IS, Fadel HE. Indications for and timing of delivery in diabetic pregnancies. Am J Obstet Gynecol. 1985;153(7):759–66.

23. Teramo K, Hiilesmaa VK. Amniotic fluid and cord plasma erythropoietin levels in pregnancies complicated by preeclampsia,

pregnancy-induced hypertension and chronic hypertension. J Perinat Med. 2004;32(3):240–7.

24. Miehle K, Stepan H. Leptin, adiponectin and other adipokines in gestational diabetes mellitus and pre-eclampsia. Clin Endocrinol. 2012;76(1):2–11.

25. Vintzileos AM, Gaffney SE. The relationship between fetal biophysical profile and cord pH in patients undergoing cesarean section before the onset of labor. Obstet Gynecol. 1987;70(2):196–201.

26. Moore TR, Piacquadio K. A prospective evaluation of fetal movement screening to reduce the incidence of antepartum fetal death. Am J Obstet Gynecol. 1989;160(5):1075–80.

27. Frøen JF, Heazell AE. Fetal movement assessment. Semin Perinatol. 2008;32(4):243–6.

28. Lagrew DC Jr. The contraction stress test. Clin Obstet Gynecol. 1995;38(1):11–25.

29. Freeman RK, Anderson G. A prospective multi-institutional study of antepartum fetal heart rate monitoring: II. Contraction stress test versus nonstress test for primary surveillance. Am J Obstet Gynecol. 1982;143(7):778–81.

30. Devoe LD. Antenatal fetal assessment: contraction stress test, nonstress test, vibroacoustic stimulation, amniotic fluid volume, biophysical profile, and modified biophysical profile — an overview. Semin Perinatol. 2008;32(4):247–52.

31. American College of Obstetrics and Gynecology. Practice bulletin no. 145: antepartum fetal surveillance. Obstet Gynecol. 2014;124(1):182–90.

32. Clark SL, Sabey P. Nonstress testing with acoustic stimulation and amniotic fluid volume assessment: 5973 tests without unexpected fetal death. Am J Obstet Gynecol. 1989;160(3): 694–7.

33. Smith CV, Phelan JP. Fetal acoustic stimulation testing: II. A randomized clinical comparison with the nonstress test. Am J Obstet Gynecol. 1986;155(1):131–4.

34. Cousins LM, Poeltler DM. Nonstress testing at ≤ 32.0 weeks' gestation: a randomized trial comparing different assessment criteria. Am J Obstet Gynecol. 2012;207(4):311.

35. Girz BA, Divon MY, Merkatz IR. Sudden fetal death in women with well-controlled, intensively monitored gestational diabetes. J Perinatol. 1992;12(3):229–33.

36. Barrett JM, Salyer SL. The nonstress test: an evaluation of 1000 patients. Am J Obstet Gynecol. 1981;141(2):153–7.

37. Pazos R, Vuolo K. Association of spontaneous fetal heart rate decelerations during antepartum nonstress testing and intrauterine growth retardation. Am J Obstet Gynecol. 1982;144(5):574–7.
38. Manning FA, Morrison I. Fetal biophysical profile scoring: selective use of the nonstress test. Am J Obstet Gynecol. 1987;156(3):709–12.
39. Miller DA, Rabello YA. The modified biophysical profile: antepartum testing in the 1990s. Am J Obstet Gynecol. 1996;174(3):812–7.
40. Nageotte MP, Towers CV. Perinatal outcome with the modified biophysical profile. Am J Obstet Gynecol. 1994;170(5):1672–6.
41. Eller DP, Stramm SL. The effect of maternal intravenous glucose administration on fetal activity. Am J Obstet Gynecol. 1992;167(4):1071–4.
42. Vintzileos AM, Campbell WA. The use and misuse of the fetal biophysical profile. Am J Obstet Gynecol. 1987;156(3):527–33.
43. Biggio JR, Wenstrom KD. Hydramnios prediction of adverse perinatal outcome. Obstet Gynecol. 1999;94(5):773–7.
44. Pilliod RA, Page JM. The risk of fetal death in nonanomalous pregnancies affected by polyhydramnios. Am J Obstet Gynecol. 2015;213(3):410–e1.
45. Salvesen DR, Freeman J. Prediction of fetal acidaemia in pregnancies complicated by maternal diabetes mellitus by biophysical profile scoring and fetal heart rate monitoring. Br J Obstet Gynaecol. 1993;100(3):227–33.
46. Johnson JM, Lange IR. Biophysical profile scoring in the management of the diabetic pregnancy. Obstet Gynecol. 1988;72(6):841–6.
47. Kjos SL, Leung A. Antepartum surveillance in diabetic pregnancies: predictors of fetal distress in labor. Am J Obstet Gynecol. 1995;173(5):1532–9.
48. Kingdom JC, Burrell SJ. Pathology and clinical implications of abnormal umbilical artery Doppler waveforms. Ultrasound Obstet Gynecol. 1997;9(4):271–86.
49. Alfirevic Z, Stampalija T. Fetal and umbilical Doppler ultrasound in high-risk pregnancies. Cochrane Libr. 2010;1(1):CD007529.
50. Berkley E, Chauhan SP. Doppler assessment of the fetus with intrauterine growth restriction. Am J Obstet Gynecol. 2012;206(4):300–8.
51. Bracero LA, Figueroa R, Byrne DW, Han HJ. Comparison of umbilical Doppler velocimetry, nonstress testing, and biophysi-

cal profile in pregnancies complicated by diabetes. J Ultrasound Med. 1996;15(4):301–8.

52. Bracero LA, Haberman S. Maternal glycemic control and umbilical artery Doppler velocimetry. J Matern Fetal Neonatal Med. 2002;12(5):342–8.

53. Wong SF, Chan FY. Use of umbilical artery Doppler velocimetry in the monitoring of pregnancy in women with pre-existing diabetes. Aust N Z J Obstet Gynaecol. 2003;43(4):302–6.

54. Reece EA, Homko CJ. Doppler velocimetry and the assessment of fetal well-being in normal and diabetic pregnancies. Ultrasound Obstet Gynecol. 1994;4(6):508–14.

55. Gutaj P, Wender-Ozegowska E. Diagnosis and management of IUGR in pregnancy complicated by type 1 diabetes mellitus. Curr Diab Rep. 2016;16(5):1–9.

56. Landon MB, Vickers S. Fetal surveillance in pregnancy complicated by diabetes mellitus: is it necessary? J Matern Fetal Neonatal Med. 2002;12(6):413–6.

57. American College of Obstetricians and Gynecologists. ACOG practice bulletin no. 134: fetal growth restriction. Obstet Gynecol. 2013;121(5):1122.

Chapter 18
Contraception for Women with Diabetes

Sushila Arya and Sanja Kupesic

Fast Facts

- Two-thirds of pregnancies in diabetic patients are unplanned.
- Combined hormonal contraceptives are safe for women with diabetes without vascular complications.
- Progestin-only contraceptives and IUDs are recommended for diabetic patients with microvascular complications and patients with contraindications to estrogen.

S. Arya, MD, FACOG (✉)
Department of Obstetrics and Gynecology, Paul L. Foster School of Medicine, Texas Tech University Health Sciences Center El Paso, 4801 Alberta Avenue, El Paso, TX 79905, USA
e-mail: Sushila.arya@ttuhsc.edu

S. Kupesic, MD, PhD
Department of Obstetrics and Gynecology, Paul L. Foster School of Medicine, Texas Tech University Health Sciences Center El Paso, 5001 El Paso Dr, El Paso, TX 79905, USA
e-mail: sanja.kupesic@ttuhsc.edu

© Springer International Publishing AG 2018   209
L.E. Moore (ed.), *Diabetes in Pregnancy*,
https://doi.org/10.1007/978-3-319-65518-5_18

18.1   Introduction

In the United States, approximately 2% of women between the ages of 20 and 39 years old have diabetes mellitus [1]. The use of contraception has been shown to reduce pregnancy-related morbidity and mortality. Certain methods may reduce the risk of reproductive cancers and may also be used to treat some menstrual-related problems. According to the 2002 National Survey of Family Growth, a total of 6.4 million pregnancies occurred during that year and half were unintended. Interestingly, 48% of the reported pregnancies occurred in couples using a contraceptive method. There is a significant association between repeated unintended pregnancies and nonuse of contraceptives [2]. Contraceptive counseling should include a discussion of failure rates and reinforcement of consistent and correct use of the method. Unintended pregnancies are most likely to occur among young, unmarried, Black, Latina, and low-income women [3]. There is no single best fit for contraceptive use. Each contraceptive method has advantages and disadvantages. With currently available methods, fertility is easily regained on discontinuation of use.

Diabetes mellitus (DM) with or without end organ involvement may be a contraindication to some contraceptive methods mainly due to increased cardiovascular and venothromboembolism risk. The World Health Organization (WHO) published detailed guidelines on medical eligibility criteria for the use of contraceptive methods. The most recent fourth edition can be downloaded from the following website: (www.who.int/reproductivehealth/publications/family_planning/9789241563888/en/index.html) [4]. The Centers for Disease Control and Prevention (CDC) guidelines, specific to practice in the United States, were published in 2010 and are available at http://www.cdc.gov/mmwr/preview/mmwrhtml/rr59e0528a1.htm [5].

Gestational diabetes mellitus (GDM) usually develops in midpregnancy and typically affects 3–10% of all pregnant women. GDM is a harbinger of future health problems, and up to 30–70% of women with GDM will develop type 2 diabetes mellitus (T2DM) [6]. Effective contraception can potentially ward off the future development of T2DM by allowing appropriate interval and healthy lifestyle changes between pregnancies [7]. Diabetes affects both maternal and fetal metabolism leading to adverse pregnancy outcomes. Pregnancy loss is significantly higher among patients with diabetes. Between 5% and 8% of diabetic mothers with poor metabolic control during the period of organogenesis are affected by birth defects which are twice the rate of the general population [8]. Pregnant patients with DM are at increased risk of preeclampsia and higher perinatal mortality [9]. Microvascular complications like retinopathy and nephropathy can deteriorate with pregnancy [10]. The fetal and maternal pregnancy outcomes can be modified with appropriate glycemic control through a healthy diet before and during conception, planned exercise programs, and lifestyle modifications [11]. Unfortunately, women with diabetes are less likely to receive contraceptive counseling or use contraception compared to women without diabetes. Almost two-thirds of pregnancies in women with diabetes are unplanned [12, 13]. Diabetic mothers are insufficiently aware of the importance of strict metabolic control with normal or near-normal glucose levels. Hence there is absolute need for improved preconception counseling.

18.2   Considerations for Women with Diabetes Mellitus

The Centers for Disease Control and Prevention has developed a Summary Chart of US Medical Eligibility Criteria (MEC) for contraceptive use. The MEC for contraceptive use chart provides recommendation for the use of contraceptive methods depending upon certain medical morbidities. Healthcare providers can utilize the chart when providing recommendations of contraceptive methods based on characteristics and medical conditions of the individual. The chart is organized into four categories. According to the chart, category 1 comprises condition, which imposes no restriction for selecting contraceptive method. Category 2 comprises medical conditions where contraceptive methods can be use but close follow-up is indicated. In category 3 the use of a particular method is not advisable, unless other method is not acceptable or available, and its prescription requires cautious clinical judgment and close follow-up. Category 4 comprises conditions that impose unacceptable risk with the use of a contraceptive method. Diabetic women with complications is category 3 if microvascular complications are present or category 4 if vascular disease or diabetes was diagnosed >20 years ago [5].

Safety and effectiveness of contraception in healthy women is well studied, but literature pertaining to their use among women with coexisting medical problems (e.g., cardiovascular disease, obesity, hypertension, lipid disorders, and DM) is relatively scarce [14]. It is known that repeat pregnancies pose a higher risk of development of T2DM when compared to the use of low-dose combined oral contraceptives (COCs) [15]. This makes postpartum education to promote breastfeeding, diet, weight management, exercise, and contraception counseling even more crucial. Use of levonorgestrel IUD (LNG-IUD) doesn't affect postpartum glucose in women with a history of GDM [16]. Also, there is no increase in the incidence of T2DM with the use of COC in women who had a prior history of GDM [17]. History of GMD is not a contraindication to any form of contraception, but associated risk factors such as hypertension, obesity, and dyslipidemia should be considered. Hormonal or nonhormonal contraception use in the postpartum period is not influenced by a history of GDM among nondiabetic primiparous women [7].

Hormonal contraception (current or past use) does not appear to precipitate the development of T2DM in healthy women [18–20]. Hormonal contraceptives are safe and effective birth control options for women who are insulin-dependent diabetics without vascular disease [21]. The use of

COCs by women with insulin-dependent DM without vascular involvement does not pose additional risk for development of early retinopathy and/or nephropathy [22]. A Cochrane review compared progestin-only, combined, and nonhormonal contraceptives and their effect on glucose and lipid metabolism and macro- and microvascular complications when used for women with type 1 DM (T1DM) [23]. The randomized control trials included in this comprehensive review were insufficient to draw definite conclusions. However, no difference was found in daily insulin requirement, HbA1c, or fasting blood glucose after 1 year of use of contraception [23]. Similarly, for women without DM, there was no significant effect on glucose metabolism or on the insulin secretion profile with the use of COCs containing ethinyl estradiol (EE) lower than 35 mcg [24, 25]. The use of high-dose COC and COC containing 30 mcg ethinyl estradiol + 75 mcg gestodene was found to cause slight impairment in glucose metabolism [23].

In systematic meta-analyses, progesterone-only COCs were not associated with increased odds of venous or arterial thrombotic events [26–28]. Therefore progesterone-only contraceptives are recommended by the World Health Organization for women with advanced diabetes or women with diabetes and other cardiovascular risk factors [4]. There is reassuring data reporting no increase in the severity of microvascular complications (retinopathy and nephropathy) in women with T1DM with the use of COC [10, 22]. However, in a Danish retrospective study, a tenfold higher risk of cerebral thromboembolism was noted in women with diabetes who were using COC [29]. Another recent study reported a fourfold increase in venous thromboembolism (VTE) with use of progestin-only pills or depot medroxyprogesterone acetate (DMPA) compared to nonuser of hormonal contraception or IUD users [30, 31]. Higher risk of stroke [32, 33] and myocardial infarction with the use of COC in women with DM was reported [34]. There is also an increased risk of stroke with the use of injectable progesterone for contraception in women with diabetes and hypertension [35]. Larger prospective studies are required to completely reveal the estrogen and progesterone effects on microvasculature. Caution should be exercised to prescribe COC specifically to diabetic women with uncontrolled microvascular complications like retinopathy or nephropathy with persistent proteinuria.

There is no significant difference in carbohydrate metabolism in women with T1DM using levonorgestrel-releasing intrauterine system (LNG-IUS) and copper IUD [23]. Intrauterine and implantable subdermal contraceptives are highly effective reversible contraceptives and have the lowest absolute risk in women with DM [31, 36].

18.3   Long-Acting Reversible Contraceptive (LARC) Methods

Intrauterine contraception should be the first choice of contraception for all women, including nulliparous and multiparous [37]. Obesity-related abnormal uterine bleeding (AUB-O) is frequently associated in patients with diabetes, and recommendations of LNG-IUS should be preferred over other contraceptives. Table 18.1 illustrates various LARC options, while Table 18.2 reviews contraindications for the use of LARC [31].

Nexplanon has been in use since 2011; it contains 68 mg of etonogestrel and prevents pregnancy for up to 3 years. It also contains barium sulfate, which makes it radiopaque. The implant continuously releases etonogestrel which prevents fertilization by inhibiting ovulation and thickening of cervical mucus. Paragard or Cu T380A contains no hormone, and its contraceptive action is by releasing copper ions into the uterine cavity, which interferes with sperm transport, fertilization, and implantation through a local inflammatory reaction. Paragard is a reliable LARC method for patients who have contraindications to the use of hormonal contraceptives. LNG-IUS works by releasing levonorgestrel which thickens the cervical mucus, alters the endometrium, and inhibits

TABLE 18.1 Various long-acting reversible contraceptive methods

Method	Irregular bleeding	Amenorrhea	Ovulation inhibition	Heavy bleeding	Failure rate	Duration (year)
Paragard	−	−	−	+/−	0.8	10
Mirena[a] (52 mg)	+/−	+/−	−	−	0.1	5
Liletta[a] (52 mg)	+/−	+/−	−	−	0.1	4
Skyla[a] (13.5 mg)	+/−	+/−	−	−	0.1	3
Subdermal implant (Nexplanon)	+/−	+/−	+	−	0.05	3

[a]Levonorgestrel-releasing intrauterine system (LNG-IUS)
Adapted from Ref. [38]

TABLE 18.2 Contraindications for use of long-acting reversible contraceptive methods

Contraindication for hormonal LARC use	Contraindication for IUD use
Unexplained vaginal bleeding	Active sexually transmitted infection
Acute DVT/PE	Anatomic abnormalities of the uterus
SLE with antiphospholipid antibodies	
Severe cirrhosis, liver tumor	
Current breast, ovarian, or endometrial cancer	

DVT deep vein thrombosis, *PE* pulmonary embolism, *SLE* systemic lupus erythematous, *IUD* intrauterine device. Adapted from World Health Organization (WHO). Medical eligibility criteria for contraceptive use. 5th edition. World Health Organization; 2015. Available at: http://www.who.int/reproductivehealth/publications/family_planning/Ex-Summ-MEC-5/en/ [4]

sperm motility and in some women ovulation. Antibiotics use is not recommended prior to IUD insertion. STI testing should be done in those with high-risk behavior. Women who test positive for gonorrhea or chlamydia at the time of insertion should be prescribed appropriate antibiotics without removing the IUD, unless the STI results in an acute PID or tubo-ovarian abscess (TOA) formation are not responding to medical management [37].

18.4   Hormonal Contraception

Over 80% of women in the United States have used hormonal contraception [38]. It provides effective protection against pregnancy with many noncontraceptive health benefits [14] and can safely be used by most women. Hormonal contraception includes estrogen-progesterone combined hormonal contraception (CHC) and progesterone-only methods.

TABLE 18.3 CHC classification depending upon the dose of estrogen, progestin, and type of progestin

First-generation CHC	Contains 50 mg of EE [39]
Second-generation CHC	Lower doses of estradiol (20, 30, or 35 mg) and norethindrone and its derivatives, including levonorgestrel as progestin [39]
Third-generation CHC	Progestins desogestrel, norgestimate, and gestodene; less androgenic than the second-generation progestins [40]
Fourth-generation CHC	Drospirenone, a derivative of spironolactone with antiandrogenic activity [41]

EE ethinyl estradiol

CHCs are available in several routes of administration including pills (monophasic and multiphasic), transdermal patches, and vaginal ring. Progesterone-only methods are Implanon, levonorgestrel IUDs (LNG-IUS), progestin-only pills, and Depo-Provera. Table 18.3 reviews different generations of CHC depending on the type and dose of estrogen and progestin.

The major adverse effects of hormonal contraception are VTE, hemorrhagic stroke, and myocardial infarction, which are strongly influenced by other factors like smoking, older age, and associated comorbidities (e.g., hypertension and DM) [42]. Overall quantification of the risks should be performed before prescribing any hormonal contraceptive method. The overall absolute risk of VTE in current oral contraceptive (OC) users is 6.29/10,000 woman-years. The VTE risk with the COC use is lowered with lower estrogen dose and shorter duration. The type of progesterone influences the VTE risk (cyproterone, drospirenone, gestodene, and desogestrel were associated with higher risk compared to levonorgestrel) [27].

Lauring et al. reported high rate of CHC use in women with medical contraindication to the use of estrogen [36]. Processes need to be improved to ensure those women with medical contraindications to estrogen-containing

TABLE 18.4 Absolute contraindications of CHC

Pregnancy
Undiagnosed uterine bleeding
Cigarette smoking in older than age 35
Uncontrolled hypertension
History of vascular disease and stroke (thromboembolism, atherosclerosis, and stroke)
Diabetes mellitus with complications
Breast cancer, endometrial cancer
Migraine headache with aura or peripheral neurologic symptoms called as classic migraine (increased risk of ischemic stroke)
Systemic disease that affects the vascular system (e.g., lupus erythematous, hyperlipidemia or diabetes with retinopathy or nephropathy)
Functional heart diseases (fluid retention caused by the increase in aldosterone could result in congestive heart failure), valvular heart disease with complications
Active liver disease
Prolactin-secreting macroadenoma (not a microadenoma)
Cholestasis and jaundice of pregnancy or jaundice with use of COC
Major surgery with prolonged immobilization

contraception, and who may be at an increased risk for cardiovascular events are being offered the safest and most effective methods [36]. Contradictory to that, Hanna et al. in their prospective cohort study on "The Contraceptive CHOICE Project" reported low prevalence of medical contraindications (2.83% in 5087 women) and supported provision of CHC without a prescription [43].

Table 18.4 reviews absolute contraindications for CHC use, while Table 18.5 explores different forms and routes for CHC.

TABLE 18.5 Different forms and route of combined hormonal contraception

Contraceptives	Remarks
COC pills	Fixed dose (monophasic) Multiphasic (biphasic, triphasic, or four phasic) combination 21 or 24 days of active pills, 7- or 4-day HFI
COC extended cycles	84 days of active pills, 7-day HFI
POPs	Also known as minipills, low-dose progestin, and no steroid break. These are suitable for women who are breastfeeding or have higher cardiovascular risk factors
Contraceptive patch	CHC patch which contains 6 mg norelgestromin and 0.75 mg EE (delivers approximately 150 mcg of norelgestromin and 20 mcg of EE per day) [44]
Vaginal ring	(NuvaRing®, Merck) contains 11.7 mg etonogestrel* and 2.7 mg EE (120 mcg of etonogestrel and 15 mcg of EE released per day). Similar VTE risk as oral CHC [45]
Depo-Provera (DMPA)	Injectable progesterone-only contraceptive. Two formulations, (1) 150 mg/ml for IM and 104/0.65 ml for SC injection. It is given every 3 months (13 weeks)

HFI hormone-free interval, *POPs* progestin-only pills

COC pills consist of estrogen and progesterone. COCs work by suppression of gonadotropins which leads to anovulation. The progestin-only pills (POPs) don't inhibit ovulation consistently; rather they work by cervical mucus thickening, alteration of the tubal motility, and changes of the endometrium. This explains their lower effectiveness.

A contraceptive skin patch has a surface area of 20 cm³; it contains 6 mg norelgestromin and 0.75 mg EE, delivering approximately 150 mcg of norelgestromin and 20 mcg of EE per day [44]. Norelgestromin, a third-generation progestin is the active metabolite of norgestimate. A single patch is applied each week for 3 weeks followed by no patch; hence the fourth week is a period of withdrawal bleeding. The mechanism of action is by inhibiting the ovulation; efficacy is lower for women who weigh more than 90 kg.

Contraceptive vaginal ring is flexible and soft, measures 54 mm in outer diameter, and contains 2.7 mg of ethinyl estradiol and 11.7 mg of etonogestrel. Etonogestrel is the biologically active metabolite of desogestrel, a third-generation progestin. Steroids pass through the vaginal epithelium. The ring is applied for 3 weeks and removed for 1 week to allow withdrawal bleeding. The vaginal ring delivers 120 mcg of etonogestrel and 15 mcg of EE. The mechanism is similar to the contraceptive patch and pills, by inhibiting ovulation, thickening the cervical mucus, and therefore decreasing the chance of fertilization.

The only injectable contraceptives available in the United States are depot medroxyprogesterone acetate (DMPA). The injection is given once every 3 months and uses 150 mg for intramuscular (IM) use or 104 mg for subcutaneous (SC) use. These formulations are crystalline suspension, which slowly release the progesterone. The IM formulation is given deeply into the gluteal or deltoid muscle. The subcutaneous formulations are for use into the SC on abdominal wall or anterior thigh.

18.5   Coitus-Related and Barrier Methods

There are no contraindication for the use of coitus-related and barrier methods of contraception in women with diabetes. Table 18.6 provides a brief summary of the coitus-related and barrier methods.

Periodic abstinence (rhythm method) is known as avoiding sexual intercourse during the menstrual cycle days when the ovum can be fertilized. In a regular ovulatory cycle, it requires abstinence for 6 days. This is based on the following facts [46]:

1. Ovulation occurs 12–16 (13 ± 2) days before the onset of subsequent menses.

TABLE 18.6 Summary of coitus-related and barrier methods

Method	Remarks on use	Effectiveness
Periodic abstinence	High motivation	13.4–47/100 woman-years
Coitus interruptus	Withdrawal is the only acceptable method to some couples. Correct and consistent use with every act of intercourse. No contraindications, no devices or cost	High failure rate from sperm present in the preejaculate and withdrawal if not performed in a timely or correct way
Diaphragm	Requires highly motivated women Lower failure rates with increasing age and duration of use. Higher UTI due to obstruction of outflow, so postcoital voiding is recommended	2.8% for continuous user and 9.8% among those who used it with intercourse
Male condom	Polyurethane condoms are thinner and may provide greater sensitivity but are associated with higher rates of slippage and breakage. For this reason most experts recommend latex condoms. Highly effective if used properly, the first-year failure rates for male condom use are between 3–6% when the woman was older than 30 compared to 8–10% failure rate in women <25 years	6-month typical-use pregnancy probabilities for polyurethane and latex group are 9–10.8% and 5.4–6.4%, respectively

(continued)

TABLE 18.6 (continued)

Method	Remarks on use	Effectiveness
Female condoms	Two types available on the market: Women's condoms & Reality Made of soft polyurethane sheath with two flexible rings. Gaining more acceptability. Female controlled. May be more effective protecting against STI	Typical use failure rate is 21%
Lactational amenorrhea method	Should be used only with exclusive breastfeeding and up to 6 months after delivery. Amenorrhea depends upon frequency, duration, and night nursing	Failure rate is 0.9–1.2% among amenorrheic and exclusively breastfeeding women

2. Ovum can be fertilized within 24 h after ovulation.
3. Fertilizing capacity of a spermatozoon lasts for 48 h after coitus.

The periodic abstinence method requires relatively long periods of abstinence; hence pregnancy rates are high with this method, ranging from 13.4 to 47/100 woman-years (Pearl Index) [46]. The practical effectiveness of this method is around 75%; meaning that about a quarter of the couples practicing it will generate a child in any given year.

Diaphragm is a thin dome-shaped membrane made of latex rubber or silicone with a flexible spring modeled in a ring. The spring allows fitting of the diaphragm well to separate the vagina from the cervix. For best effectiveness of this method, the physician has to find the accurate size for an individual patient. Diaphragms were the most widely used female-controlled reversible contraceptive method prior to the introduction of oral contraceptive. Diaphragms should be used with spermicide and left in place for 8 h after the last coital act. The failure rate varies depending on its continuous use vs. use with intercourse act. In a nonrandomized study, the failure rate was 2.8% among women who left the diaphragm in place without using spermicide. They removed it only during menses and once daily to wash it followed by immediate reinsertion. On the other hand, the 12-month failure rate was much higher, 9.8% among women who used it with a spermicide in the usual manner (with sexual intercourse and then leaving it in for 8 h thereafter). Diaphragm is inexpensive and reversible method of contraception but requires placement before sexual activity. Clearly, its effectiveness depends on patient motivation, skill, and experience.

FDA-approved male condoms are made of either latex or polyurethane.

Physicians should encourage use of condoms especially to individuals with multiple sex partners to prevent both pregnancy and the transmission of sexually transmitted infections. Clinicians should educate both men and women about the proper use of condoms; the following website provides detailed instructions: www.plannedparenthood.org/health-topics/birthcontrol/condom10187.htm

The female condoms are made of soft polyurethane sheath with two flexible rings. The inner ring, which lies at the closed end, serves as an internal anchor for the condom, and the outer ring forms the external edge of the device and remains outside the vagina. Female condom has few advantages over male condoms. The polyurethane used in female condoms is thicker than latex or polyurethane used in male condoms so it is less likely to rupture. This contraception is female controlled, and by covering the external genital, it provides greater STI protection. Women's condoms and Reality are two types of female condoms available worldwide. Since 2004 Women's condoms have been found to be acceptable, safe, and excellent in performance through various clinical studies [47–50]. A comprehensive Cochrane review of various studies comparing the female condom to male condoms reported that female condoms are as effective in STI and unwanted pregnancy prevention as male condoms [51]. Mathematical model researchers have calculated that with consistent female condom use, the HIV transmission can be reduced to 90% compared to unprotected intercourse [52].

Lactational amenorrhea method (LAM): elevated prolactin during breastfeeding inhibits gonadotropin pulsatility and causes amenorrhea. The amenorrhea lasts for a variable length of time depending upon frequency and duration of nursing. Night nursing is specifically associated with anovulation and amenorrhea. This method should be used only with exclusive breastfeeding and up to 6 months after delivery. The cumulative pregnancy rate among fully breast-feeding, amenorrheic women who are not using any other contraceptive method was noted to be 0.9–1.2. This may underestimate the risk, as rates of sexual activity may be lower in many postpartum women.

18.6   Female Sterilization

There are several different techniques of occluding fallopian tubes that are used for permanent contraception in women. Female sterilization is the most common contraception method used worldwide and second most common contraceptive method used in the United States [53]. Female sterilization is a highly effective method of contraception with less than <1% risk of pregnancy after sterilization [54].

There is no strict medical contraindication to sterilization; however, various medical conditions (e.g., morbid obesity and significant risk factors for intra-abdominal adhesions) might influence the preferred route of female sterilization, and medical comorbidities (cardiac, pulmonary, renal, or neurologic dysfunction) will increase the anesthesia risk.

Sterilization can be done laparoscopically (tubal occlusion by electrosurgical desiccation or mechanical methods like silicone band, titanium clip, or spring clip), hysteroscopically (Essure), or via minilaparotomy (abdominal postpartum sterilization). Essure is the only hysteroscopic sterilization device approved by FDA in 2002 and available in the United States. Essure is a micro-insert system made of polymer and metal and measures 4 cm in length and 1–2 mm wide.

Before any route or technique of female sterilization, the following should be accomplished:

1. Counseling about alternatives, types, efficacy, and permanency of female sterilization.
2. Assessment or risk factors for regret.
3. Preoperative surgical risk assessment, appropriate testing, and thorough consultation.
4. Pregnancy test and use of a reliable contraceptive method until sterilization procedure is complete.
5. Informed consent after thorough discussion of risk, benefits, and alternatives about the chosen sterilization procedure. (The US federal sterilization consent requires obtaining informed consent between 30–180 days prior to the procedure; however, state and institutional policies may differ.)

18.7   Emergency Contraception

Pregnancy should always be ruled out before using any emergency contraceptive method. Emergency contraceptive should be started as soon as possible after unprotected intercourse. Hormonal emergency contraceptives are less effective for patients with higher BMI, and the effectiveness decreases as the interval after unprotected intercourse increases, especially if used later than 72 h after intercourse. Table 18.7 lists methods of emergency contraception, side effects, and the window of time for use after unprotected intercourse.

TABLE 18.7 Various methods of emergency contraception

Method	Window[a]	Side effects	Remarks
Copper IUD	7	Usual IUD related insertion issues	Most effective emergency contraceptive method
Ulipristal acetate 30 mg	5	Nausea and vomiting	Not effective if used on day of ovulation or after ovulation
LNG 1.5 mg (Plan B One-Step)	5	Nausea and vomiting	Highly effective if used before ovulation

[a]Window: to be used within this period after unprotected intercourse
LNG levonorgestrel. Adapted from Ref. [55]

18.8   Conclusion

At this time ACOG recommends that the use of COC in women with diabetes should be limited to patients younger than 35 years who do not smoke and are otherwise healthy, with no evidence of hypertension, nephropathy, retinopathy, or other vascular disease [13]. Women with diabetes should be encouraged to utilize effective and safe contraceptive methods depending upon their risk factors and need of contraception. LARCs are highly effective and have higher continuation rate and can be used by most women with diabetes. Table 18.8 reviews medical eligibility criteria for the use of COC and POP in women with DM.

18.9   Future of Male Contraception

Vasectomy is a surgical sterilization option available for couples who are in a lifelong relationship in which a female partner may or may not have an underlying condition that is restricting the use of an alternative female contraception method. More recently temporary vasectomy (vasovagal)

TABLE 18.8 Medical eligibility criteria for combined oral contraceptives and progestin-only pills in women with DM

Type of DM	COC and progestin-only pills
History of GDM	No restrictions. General risk factors should be reviewed
Type I or II DM (absence of microvascular complications)	Advantage outweighs the risk
Microvascular complications (retinopathy, nephropathy, neuropathy)	Unacceptable health risk with COC but with POP advantage outweighs the risk Nonhormonal contraception should be preferred [55]
Other vascular disease or DM >20 years	Unacceptable health risk with COC but with POP advantage outweighs the risk Nonhormonal contraception should be preferred [55]

Adapted from Refs [4, 5]

was developed, involving a gel injection into the vas deferens. Reversibility is achieved by flushing the gel at any point if the man changes his mind. A male contraceptive implant called MENT is currently undergoing a clinical trial in Europe. The device releases a synthetic steroid that resembles testosterone affecting sperm cell development. There have been minimal side effects, and no effects on the libido, bone loss, and/or bone mass are encouraging the progress of phase 2 clinical trials. Similar results are achieved with contraceptive gels containing testosterone or progestins. The gels are rubbed onto the skin leading to inhibition of the sperm production. Major advantages of this method are reversibility of this contraceptive method and a quick return to normal sperm count after stopping its use. The search for a male contraceptive pill not associated with major side effects is on its way. Multiple hormonal and nonhormonal methods of male contraception are in the drug developmental stages, with the hope that a reversible, reliable, and a safe method of male contraception will be available to couples soon [56].

References

1. Cowie CC, Rust KF, Byrd-Holt DD, Eberhardt MS, Flegal KM, Engelgau MM, et al. Prevalence of diabetes and impaired fasting glucose in adults in the U.S. population: National Health and Nutrition Examination Survey 1999-2002. Diabetes Care. 2006;29(6):1263–8.
2. Matsuda Y, Masho S, McGrath JM. The relationship between repeated unintended pregnancies and current contraceptive use: National Survey of Family Growth (NSFG) 2006–2008 data. J Community Health Nurs. 2012;29:163–72.
3. Chandra A, Martinez GM, Mosher WD, Abma JC, Jones J. Fertility, family planning, and reproductive health of U.S. women: data from the 2002 National Survey of Family Growth. Vital Health Stat. 2005;23(25):1–160.
4. Powers BJ, Brown G, Williams RW, Speers W. Medical eligibility criteria for contraceptive use. World Heal Organ. 2015;87(5):276. Available from: http://link.springer.com/10.2165/00128413-200112870-00010%5Cn, http://www.ncbi.nlm.nih.gov/pubmed/1519579
5. Medical Eligibility Criteria for Contraceptive Use. Adapted from the World Health Organization Medical Eligibility Criteria for Contraceptive Use, MMWR, vol. 59, 4th ed. Recommendations and reports: Morbidity and mortality weekly report. Recommendations and reports/Centers for Disease Control. 2010. p. 1–86. Available from: http://ovidsp.ovid.com/ovidweb.cgi?T=JS&PAGE=reference&D=emed9&NEWS=N&AN=20559203.
6. Kim C, Newton KM, Knopp RH. Gestational diabetes and the incidence of type 2 diabetes. Diabetes Care. 2002;25(10):7.
7. Beydoun HA, Beydoun MA, Tamim H. How does gestational diabetes affect postpartum contraception in nondiabetic primiparous women? Contraception. 2009;79(4):290–6.
8. Weintrob N, Karp M, Moshe H. Short- and long-range complications in offspring of diabetic mothers. J Diabetes Complicat. 1996;10(5):294–301.
9. Ng CHM, Fraser IS, Berbic M. Contraception for women with medical disorders. Best Pract Res Clin Obstet Gynaecol. 2014;28(6):917–30.
10. Klein BEK, Klein R, Moss SE. Exogenous estrogen exposures and changes in diabetic retinopathy: the Wisconsin epidemiologic study of diabetic retinopathy. Diabetes Care. 1999;22(12):1984–7.

11. Kjaer K, Hagen C, Sando SH, Eshoj O. Contraception in women with IDDM: an epidemiological study. Diabetes Care. 1992;15(11):1585–90.
12. Diabetes Care. Standards of medical care in diabetes—2016: summary of revisions. Diabetes Care. 2016;39(Suppl 1):S4–5. Available from: http://www.ncbi.nlm.nih.gov/pubmed/26696680%5Cnhttp://care.diabetesjournals.org/lookup/doi/10.2337/dc16-S003
13. Vahratian A, Barber JS, Lawrence JM, Kim C. Family-planning practices among women with diabetes and overweight and obese women in the 2002 National Survey for Family Growth. Diabetes Care. 2009;32(6):1026–31.
14. Kaunitz A. ACOG practice bulletin no. 73: use of hormonal contraception in women with coexisting medical conditions. Obstet Gynecol. 2006;107(6):1453–72. Available from: http://www.ncbi.nlm.nih.gov/pubmed/16738183
15. Kjos SL. After pregnancy complicated by diabetes: postpartum care and education. Obstet Gynecol Clin N Am. 2007;34:335–49.
16. Kiley JW, Hammond C, Niznik C, Rademaker A, Liu D, Shulman LP. Postpartum glucose tolerance in women with gestational diabetes using levonorgestrel intrauterine contraception. Contraception. 2015;91(1):67–70.
17. Kjos SL, Peters RK, Xiang A, Thomas D, Schaefer U, Buchanan TA. Contraception and the risk of type 2 diabetes mellitus in Latina women with prior gestational diabetes mellitus. JAMA. 1998;280(6):533–8. Available from: http://www.ncbi.nlm.nih.gov/pubmed/9707143
18. Kim C, Siscovick DS, Sidney S, Lewis CE, Kiefe CI, Koepsell TD. Oral contraceptive use and association with glucose, insulin, and diabetes in young adult women: the CARDIA study. Diabetes Care. 2002;25(6):1027–32. Available from: http://care.diabetesjournals.org/content/25/6/1027.full
19. Chasan-Taber L, Willett WC, Stampfer MJ, Hunter DJ, Colditz GA, Spiegelman D, et al. A prospective study of oral contraceptives and NIDDM among U.S. women. Diabetes care. 1997;20(3):330–5. Available from: http://www.ncbi.nlm.nih.gov/pubmed/9051382
20. Rimm EB, Manson JE, Stampfer MJ, Colditz GA, Willett WC, Rosner B, et al. Oral contraceptive use and the risk of type 2 (non-insulin-dependent) diabetes mellitus in a large prospective study of women. Diabetologia. 1992;35(10):967–72.
21. Gourdy P. Diabetes and oral contraception. Best Pract Res Clin Endocrinol Metab. 2013;27(1):67–76.

22. Garg SK, Chase HP, Marshall G, Hoops SL, Holmes DL, Jackson WE. Oral contraceptives and renal and retinal complications in young women with insulin-dependent diabetes mellitus. JAMA. 1994;271(14):1099–102. Available from: http://www.ncbi.nlm.nih. gov/pubmed/8151852

23. Visser J, Snel M, Van Vliet Huib AAM. Hormonal versus non-hormonal contraceptives in women with diabetes mellitus type 1 and 2. Cochrane Database Syst Rev. 2013;(3):CD003990. doi: 10.1002/14651858.CD003990.pub4. Review. PMID: 23543528.

24. Sitruk-Ware R, Nath A. Metabolic effects of contraceptive steroids. Rev Endocr Metab Disord. 2011;12(2):63–75.

25. Lopez LM, Grimes DA, Schulz KF. Steroidal contraceptives: effect on carbohydrate metabolism in women without diabetes mellitus. Cochrane Database Syst Rev. 2007;(2):CD006133.

26. Tepper NK, Whiteman MK, Marchbanks PA, James AH, Curtis KM. Progestin-only contraception and thromboembolism: a systematic review. Contraception. 2016;94:678–700.

27. Lidegaard O, Lokkegaard E, Svendsen AL, Agger C. Hormonal contraception and risk of venous thromboembolism: national follow-up study. BMJ. 2009;339:b2890. Available from: http:// www.bmj.com/content/339/bmj.b2890.full.pdf+html

28. Mantha S, Karp R, Raghavan V, Terrin N, Bauer KA, Zwicker JI. Assessing the risk of venous thromboembolic events in women taking progestin-only contraception: a meta-analysis. BMJ. 2012;345(aug07 2):e4944. Available from: http://www.bmj. com/cgi/doi/10.1136/bmj.e4944

29. Lidegaard O. Oral-contraceptives, pregnancy and the risk of cerebral thromboembolism - the influence of diabetes, hypertension, migraine and previous thrombotic disease. Br J Obstet Gynaecol. 1995;102(2):153–9.

30. Van Hylckama VA, Helmerhorst FM, Rosendaal FR. The risk of deep venous thrombosis associated with injectable depot-medroxyprogesterone acetate contraceptives or a levonorgestrel intrauterine device. Arterioscler Thromb Vasc Biol. 2010;30(11):2297–300.

31. O'Brien SH, Koch T, Vesely SK, Schwarz EB. Hormonal contraception and risk of thromboembolism in women with diabetes. Diabetes Care. 2017;40(2):233–8.

32. Petitti DB, Sidney S, Bernstein A, Wolf S, Quesenberry C, Ziel HK. Stroke in users of low-dose oral contraceptives. N Engl J Med. 1996;335(1):8–15. Available from: pm:8637557

33. Contraception SH. Ischaemic stroke and combined oral contraceptives: results of an international, multicentre, case-control study. WHO collaborative study of cardiovascular disease and steroid hormone contraception. Lancet. 1996;348(9026):498–505. Available from: http://www.ncbi.nlm.nih.gov/pubmed/8757151

34. Tanis BC, van den Bosch MA, Kemmeren JM, Cats VM, Helmerhorst FM, Algra A, et al. Oral contraceptives and the risk of myocardial infarction. N Engl J Med. 2001;345(25):1787–93. Available from: http://www.ncbi.nlm.nih.gov/pubmed/11752354

35. World Health Organization. Cardiovascular disease and use of oral and injectable progestogen-only contraceptives and combined injectable contraceptives - results of an international, multicenter, case-control study. Contraception. 1998;57(5):315–24.

36. Lauring JR, Lehman EB, Deimling TA, Legro RS, Chuang CH. Combined hormonal contraception use in reproductive-age women with contraindications to estrogen use. Am J Obstet Gynecol. 2016;215(3):330.e1–7. Available from: http://dx.doi.org/10.1016/j.ajog.2016.03.047

37. Black A, Guilbert E, Costescu D, Dunn S, Fisher W, Kives S, et al. Canadian contraception consensus (part 3 of 4): chapter 7 - intrauterine contraception. J Obstet Gynaecol Can. 2016;38(2):182–222.

38. Daniels K, Mosher WD. Contraceptive methods women have ever used: United States, 1982–2010. Natl Health Stat Report. 2013;(62):1–15. Available from: http://www.ncbi.nlm.nih.gov/pubmed/24988816

39. Lewis MA. The transnational study on oral contraceptives and the health of young women. Methods, results, new analyses and the healthy user effect. Hum Reprod Update. 1999;5(6):707–20.

40. Speroff L, DeCherney A. Evaluation of a new generation of oral contraceptives. The advisory board for the new progestins. Obstet Gynecol. 1993;81:1034–47.

41. Muhn P, Fuhrmann U, Fritzemeier KH, Krattenmacher R, Schillinger E. Drospirenone: a novel progestogen with antimineralocorticoid and antiandrogenic activity. Ann N Y Acad Sci. 1995;761:311–35.

42. Farley TM, Collins J, Schlesselman JJ. Hormonal contraception and risk of cardiovascular disease. An international perspective. Contraception. 1998;57(3):211–30. Available from: http://www.ncbi.nlm.nih.gov/pubmed/9617537

43. Xu H, Eisenberg DL, Madden T, Secura GM, Peipert JF. Medical contraindications in women seeking combined hormonal contraception. Am J Obstet Gynecol. 2014;210:210.e1.

44. Abrams LS, Skee DM, Natarajan J, Wong FA, Lasseter KC. Multiple-dose pharmacokinetics of a contraceptive patch in healthy women participants. Contraception. 2001;64(5): 287–94.

45. Pfeifer S, et al. Combined hormonal contraception and the risk of venous thromboembolism: a guideline. Fertil Steril. 2017;107(1):43–51. Available from: http://linkinghub.elsevier. com/retrieve/pii/S0015028216628479

46. Jensen JT, Mishell DR Jr. Family planning contraception, sterlizaton, and pregnancy termination. In: Comprehensive Gynecology. Philadelphia: Mosby-Elsevier; 2012. p. 215–72.

47. Coffey PS, Kilbourne-Brook M, Austin G, Seamans Y, Cohen J. Short-term acceptability of the PATH Woman's condom among couples at three sites. Contraception. 2006;73(6):588–93.

48. Schwartz JL, Barnhart K, Creinin MD, Poindexter A, Wheeless A, Kilbourne-Brook M, et al. Comparative crossover study of the PATH Woman's condom and the FC female condom. Contraception. 2008;78(6):465–73.

49. Joanis C, Beksinska M, Hart C, Tweedy K, Linda J, Smit J. Three new female condoms: which do South-African women prefer? Contraception. 2011;83(3):248–54.

50. Beksinska ME, Piaggio G, Smit JA, Wu J, Zhang Y, Pienaar J, et al. Performance and safety of the second-generation female condom (FC2) versus the Woman's, the VA worn-of-women, and the Cupid female condoms: A randomised controlled non-inferiority crossover trial. Lancet Glob Health. 2013;1(3):e146.

51. Weller SC, Davis-Beaty K. Condom effectiveness in reducing heterosexual HIV transmission. Cochrane Database of Systematic Reviews 2002;(1):CD003255. doi: 10.1002/14651858.CD003255.

52. Trussell J, Sturgen K, Strickler J, Dominik R. Comparative contraceptive efficacy of the female condom and other barrier methods. Fam Plan Perspect. 1994;26(2):66–72. Available from: http://www.ncbi.nlm.nih.gov/pubmed/8033980

53. Daniels K, Daugherty J, Jones J. Current contraceptive status among women aged 15-44: United States, 2011-2013. NCHS Data Brief. 2014;173:1–8.

54. Peterson HB, Xia Z, Hughes JM, Wilcox LS, Tylor LR, Trussell J, et al. The risk of pregnancy after tubal sterilization: findings from

the U.S. collaborative review of sterilization. Am J Obstet Gynecol. 1996;174:1161–70.

55. Shawe J, Lawrenson R. Hormonal contraception in women with diabetes mellitus: Special considerations. Treat Endocrinol. 2003;2:321–30.

56. Roth MY, Page ST, Bremner WJ. Male hormonal contraception: Looking back and moving forward. Andrology. 2016;4:4–12.

Chapter 19
Diabesity

Lisa E. Moore

Fast Facts

- Obese women have increased risk of cesarean delivery.
- Maternal obesity and diabetes are risk factors for childhood obesity and early onset type 2 diabetes in offspring.
- Obesity with or without diabetes is a risk factor for congenital anomalies.

19.1 Introduction

Diabesity is obesity-dependent diabetes. It is projected that by 2030, there will be a 73% increase in adult diabetes in developing countries. In the United States, 34.9% of adults were categorized as obese in 2012 [1]. There was a 70% increase in prepregnancy obesity in the 10-year period between 1994 and 2003 [2]. One major impact of this obesity

L.E. Moore, MD, FACOG
Department of Obstetrics and Gynecology,
Texas Tech University Health Sciences Center El Paso,
Paul L. Foster School of Medicine, El Paso, TX, USA
e-mail: lisa.e.moore@ttuhsc.edu

© Springer International Publishing AG 2018
L.E. Moore (ed.), *Diabetes in Pregnancy*,
https://doi.org/10.1007/978-3-319-65518-5_19

235

trend will be the increased incidence of type 2 diabetes and the associated long-term complications. It can also be anticipated that this will lead to an increase in the number of patients who experience diabetes during pregnancy.

Using the definition of the World Health Organization, obesity is defined as a body mass index (BMI) ≥ 30 kg/m. During pregnancy, obesity is associated with increased maternal and fetal risk including hypertension, thromboembolic disease, intrapartum complications, poor wound healing, difficult intubation or difficulty placing regional anesthesia, and fetal congenital anomalies [3–5].

The "thrifty phenotype" hypothesis was proposed by Hales et al. [6] According to this theory, during human evolution, resources were either scarce or the ability to acquire those resources required significant energy expenditure. Until recently, farming and animal husbandry were labor and time intensive occupations. Humans would have evolved to utilize scarce nutrients with the expectation of a significant output of energy. This has now been altered. Today we go to the supermarket to get meat and vegetables and our lifestyles are mostly sedentary. This translates into an epidemic of excessive nutrition.

It isn't only adults who are affected. The Generation R Study [7] showed that maternal obesity was significantly associated with childhood obesity and elevated systolic blood pressure in the offspring.

19.2   Is there a Link Between Maternal Obesity and Childhood Obesity?

Obesity thresholds in childhood vary by age and gender. In the United States, childhood obesity is defined as a BMI at or above the 95th percentile for gender and age. Overweight is defined as between the 85th and 94th percentiles based on Center for Disease Control and Prevention (CDC) growth charts. The World Health Organization also produces growth charts which are used in other countries.

Maternal prepregnancy weight correlates well with fetal growth. The offspring of women who are obese or overweight at the beginning of pregnancy have a higher risk of macrosomia which is associated with an increased risk of obesity later in life. There is also evidence to indicate that infants of obese women have higher body fat and an atherogenic lipid profile. Maternal weight gain during pregnancy is positively associated with childhood and adolescent obesity in the offspring.

Importantly, these observational data points do not address causality. Certainly, there may be a genetic component, but it is also possible that environmental factors play a major role. Obese women may have poor diets which may be by choice or due to economics. The children are fed the same poor diet, thus perpetuating the cycle of obesity.

Animal studies provide the opportunity to compare genetically identical subjects and to control diet and timing of exposure. Studies in rats and sheep show that excess nutrition during pregnancy programs the offspring for obesity. These studies also indicate that a high-fat maternal diet may correlate with obesity in the offspring even when the mother does not gain weight [8]. These experiments appear to indicate that exposure during pregnancy is a critical time period for the risk of obesity. Maternal diet prior to conception, during breastfeeding, and after weaning has not been shown to be correlated with the same degree of risk.

19.3   Hypertensive Disease

Insulin resistance has been implicated in the pathogenesis of essential hypertension, ischemic heart disease, and of course type 2 diabetes. When these diseases are found in conjunction with obesity, it is termed metabolic syndrome.

The mechanisms underlying the development of pre-eclampsia and gestational hypertension in relationship to insulin resistance is unclear. Abnormal invasion of the spiral arteries results in abnormal placentation. Hyperinsulinemia and insulin resistance may potentiate this process. In the late

1990s, Sibai published a multicenter trial showing that the rate of preeclampsia was increased by 20% in women above their ideal body weight [9].

One systematic review showed that a BMI > 35 doubled the risk of preeclampsia [10].

A meta-analysis of 13 cohort studies found that the risk of preeclampsia doubled with each 5–7 point increase in pre-pregnancy BMI [11].

19.4   Gestational Diabetes

Carbohydrate intolerance is worsened during pregnancy by the normal physiologic processes in which resistance to insulin is increased. In patients with existing insulin resistance due to a higher than optimal BMI, the additional resistance to insulin may result in gestational diabetes.

19.5   Miscarriage

Obesity alone is associated with an increased risk of first trimester loss and recurrent (>3) pregnancy loss.

A matched case-control study compared women with a BMI > 30 to women with a normal BMI (19–24.9). Early (6–12 weeks), late (12–24 weeks), and recurrent (>3) miscarriages were evaluated. Four patients in the obese group were diabetic and none in the normal weight group. The study found that obesity was associated with an increased risk of first trimester loss and recurrent miscarriage [12]. These findings were confirmed by a systematic review of six studies in which the miscarriage rate in obese women was 13.6% vs 10.7% in nonobese women. There was also a higher rate of recurrent early miscarriage (0.4% vs 0.1%) [13].

An interesting study looked at underweight, overweight and obesity, and the risk of miscarriage in women with a history of recurrent loss. They found that overweight women had similar outcomes to women with ideal body weights. Both underweight and obese women had a small increased risk of miscarriage (OR, 3.98 and 1.71, respectively) [14].

19.6   Congenital Anomalies

In women with a BMI > 30, after controlling for diabetes, studies have consistently demonstrated an increased risk of heart defects, neural tube defects, limb reduction anomalies, diaphragmatic hernia, and omphalocele [15]. At least one study has demonstrated a linear relationship with increasing BMI and risk of neural tube defects [16].

A high BMI may significantly limit the efficacy of prenatal ultrasound diagnosis of anomalies. A retrospective study found that in patients with a BMI > 30, there was a nearly 50% increase in failure to adequately visualize cardiac anatomy and a 31% increase in suboptimal visualization of the intracranial and spinal anatomy [17].

19.7   Stillbirth

The pathophysiology of stillbirth in diabetic pregnancies is poorly understood.

The November 2015 MBRRACE-UK (Mothers and Babies: Reducing Risk through Audits and Confidential Enquiries across the UK) listed maternal diabetes and obesity as having an adjusted odds ratio of stillbirth of 2.5 and 1.7, respectively. One quarter of women with a stillbirth were either underweight, overweight, or obese. Half of the cases reviewed had risk factors for gestational diabetes but had not been tested.

A Danish study provides indirect evidence that strict control of blood glucose may reduce the risk of stillbirth. From 1993 to 1999, the rate of stillbirth in Denmark was 20 per 1000 deliveries. The average HA1C in patients with any poor outcome was 7.1% compared to an HA1C of 6.7% in women with uncomplicated pregnancies [18].

There is no evidence to support a specific method of antenatal testing in diabetic pregnancies to reduce the risk of stillbirth. An evaluation of growth every 3–4 weeks and weekly or twice weekly antenatal testing are common methods of surveillance.

19.8 Labor Dystocia

Obesity may alter parturition signaling in the cervix and myometrium. Obese women have longer labors, require more oxytocin, and are more likely to be diagnosed with failure to progress [19].

The Consortium on Safe Labor evaluated 228,668 deliveries in 19 hospitals between 2002 and 2008. They found that labor progressed more slowly as BMI increased.

The time from 4 to 10 cm dilation in nulliparous women was 5.4 h for BMI < 25 and 7.7 h in patients with a BMI ≥ 40. In multiparous patients with a BMI < 25, the time was 4.6 h, and in those with a BMI ≥ 40, it took a mean of 5.4 h [20].

A prospective cohort study at the University of North Carolina in which prepregnancy BMI was used to stratify term nulliparous women into normal weight (BMI < 26), overweight (BMI 26–29), and obese (BMI > 29) found that overweight and obese women, in comparison to normal weight women, received oxytocin more often and were more likely to be delivered by cesarean section, and if delivered by cesarean section, it was more likely to occur in the first stage of labor which was attributed either to fetal distress or labor dystocia. They also found that there was a longer duration of labor from 4 to 10 cm dilation [21].

19.9 Cesarean Section

Obese women are at increased risk of delivery by cesarean section. This may be due to difficulty monitoring the fetus during labor, difficulty of cervical examinations, or physicians' discomfort with the possibility of macrosomia or tissue dystocia. One study looking at more than 24,000 primiparous women found a cesarean rate of 42.6% in women with a BMI ≥ 35 compared to 14.3% in women with a BMI < 19.8 [22].

Cesarean delivery in obese women is associated with increased morbidity. In a study of the data in the Maternal-Fetal Medicine Unit Cesarean Registry, obese (BMI 30–45) and extremely obese (BMI > 45) women were at increased risk of wound infection, wound opening, and hospital readmission for a wound-related cause [23]. In contrast, using the same data, there was no increased risk of intraoperative complications [24]. Secondary analysis of the same data indicates that women with "super obesity" (BMI ≥ 50) are at increased risk of ICU admission after cesarean delivery [25].

A high BMI is directly correlated with a longer delivery to decision interval and failure of regional anesthesia in emergency cesarean deliveries. In a study from Finland, failure of regional anesthesia during an emergency cesarean was 3.7% for BMI < 30, 6.8% for BMI 30–35, and 8.5% for BMI > 35 [26]. Failure was defined as postoperative complaint of pain during cesarean section, conversion to general anesthesia, or the requirement for placing new regional anesthesia in the OR. In this study delays in the decision to delivery interval were associated with anesthesia failures, and the mean time was 33 min in the BMI < 30 group and 38 min in the BMI > 35 group.

19.10   Thromboembolism

Obese women are at increased risk of developing pulmonary embolism, and women who are either overweight or obese have an increased risk of recurrent venous thrombosis.

The National Institute for Health and Care Excellence (NICE) guidelines for postpartum care recommend that women with a BMI ≥ 30 should ambulate as soon as possible after delivery to reduce the risk. Women with a BMI ≥ 40 should be offered thromboprophylaxis.

19.11   Prematurity

Obesity is associated with iatrogenic prematurity but not spontaneous preterm birth.

A retrospective study of 14,183 patients in which mother/infant dyads were stratified based on BMI found that obese and morbidly obese women were more likely to deliver prematurely, but when complications such as hypertension, diabetes, anemia, and smoking were controlled, the rate of prematurity was not increased [27].

Palatnik et al. found that women with a high BMI had a longer cervical length during the midtrimester than women at ideal weight and a corresponding reduced rate of spontaneous preterm birth [4].

19.12   Induction of Labor

One of the most interesting findings is that obese women are less likely to experience spontaneous labor by 42 weeks. Denison found that at a BMI ≥ 35, the probability of spontaneous labor by 42 weeks was less than 50% [28]. Other studies have shown that women with a BMI > 30 were more likely to require postdates induction, and elevated BMI is a risk factor for induction of labor in nulliparous patients.

19.13   Bariatric Surgery

Bariatric surgery is typically offered to patients with a BMI ≥ 35 who have significant comorbidities which may include cardiovascular compromise or poorly controlled diabetes. More than 80% of all patients undergoing bariatric surgery are female, and in 2004, one half of all procedures were performed in reproductive-aged women [2, 29].

Bariatric surgery procedures are usually described as fitting into three categories: malabsorptive procedures that encourage weight loss by restricting absorption of nutrients, restrictive procedures that reduce the stomach capacity, and combined malabsorptive and restrictive procedures that reduce the stomach capacity and the absorptive capacity. Malabsorptive procedures are less commonly used due to long-term complications. In the United States, the most common procedures are those that reduce the stomach capacity (e.g., sleeve gastrectomy or gastric banding).

After bariatric surgery the rate of unintended pregnancy is high. A number of factors are operative; there is improved fertility with weight loss and oral medications may be poorly absorbed.

Comparisons between women who became pregnant after bariatric surgery and obese women who had not had surgery show that gestational diabetes, hypertensive disease, and fetal macrosomia occurred significantly less often in women who had bariatric surgery. There was no difference in the rate of cesarean delivery, preterm delivery, and postpartum hemorrhage. Small for gestational age was more common in the bariatric surgery group [30, 31].

19.14   Weight Gain During Pregnancy

Weight gain during pregnancy affects both the maternal and fetal health. Intra-pregnancy weight gain is associated with retention of weight postpartum and with fetal macrosomia. In a study of pregnant Danish women who were obese but not diabetic, a weight gain of 10–14.9 kg (22–32.8 lbs) was associated with increased development of hypertension, increased risk of induction of labor, and increased risk of cesarean delivery and of birthweight >4000 g [32]. The Institute of Medicine recommends that women with a BMI $\geq$ 30 should gain between 11 and 20 lbs (5–9.1 kg). In twin gestations this amount is increased to 25–42 lbs (11.3–19.1 kg) [33].

19.15   Summary

Obesity during pregnancy is associated with a number of adverse pregnancy outcomes including gestational diabetes, thromboembolism, miscarriage, congenital anomalies, stillbirth, and dysfunctional labor. The most effective treatment is prevention. Weight loss prior to pregnancy should be encouraged.

References

1. Kominiarek MA, Chauhan SP. Obesity before, during, and after pregnancy: a review and comparison of five National Guidelines. Am J Perinatol. 2016;33(5):433–41. doi:10.1055/s-0035-1567856.
2. American College of Obstetricians and Gynecologists. ACOG practice bulletin no. 105: bariatric surgery and pregnancy. Obstet Gynecol. 2009;113(6):1405–13. doi:10.1097/AOG.0b013e3181ac0544.
3. Santangeli L, Sattar N, Huda SS. Impact of maternal obesity on perinatal and childhood outcomes. Best Pract Res Clin Obstet Gynaecol. 2015;29(3):438–48. doi:10.1016/j.bpobgyn.2014.10.009.
4. Palatnik A, Miller ES, Son M, Kominiarek MA. Association among maternal obesity, cervical length, and preterm birth. Am J Perinatol. 2017;34(5):471–9. doi:10.1055/s-0036-1593350.
5. Liat S, Cabero L, Hod M, Yogev Y. Obesity in obstetrics. Best Pract Res Clin Obstet Gynaecol. 2015;29(1):79–90. doi:10.1016/j.bpobgyn.2014.05.010.
6. Hales CN, Barker DJ. Type 2 (non-insulin-dependent) diabetes mellitus: the thrifty phenotype hypothesis. Diabetologia. 1992;35(7):595–601.
7. Gaillard R, Felix JF, Duijts L, Jaddoe VW. Childhood consequences of maternal obesity and excessive weight gain during pregnancy. Acta Obstet Gynecol Scand. 2014;93(11):1085–9. doi:10.1111/aogs.12506.
8. Oken E. Maternal and child obesity: the causal link. Obstet Gynecol Clin N Am. 2009;36(2):361–77, ix-x. doi:10.1016/j.ogc.2009.03.007.
9. Sibai BM, Gordon T, Thom E, Caritis SN, Klebanoff M, McNellis D, Paul RH. Risk factors for preeclampsia in healthy nulliparous women: a prospective multicenter study. The National Institute of Child Health and Human Development Network of Maternal-Fetal Medicine Units. Am J Obstet Gynecol. 1995;172(2 Pt 1):642–8.
10. Duckitt K, Harrington D. Risk factors for pre-eclampsia at antenatal booking: systematic review of controlled studies. BMJ. 2005;330(7491):565. doi:10.1136/bmj.38380.674340.E0.
11. O'Brien TE, Ray JG, Chan WS. Maternal body mass index and the risk of preeclampsia: a systematic overview. Epidemiology. 2003;14(3):368–74.
12. Lashen H, Fear K, Sturdee DW. Obesity is associated with increased risk of first trimester and recurrent miscarriage:

matched case-control study. Hum Reprod. 2004;19(7):1644–6. doi:10.1093/humrep/deh277.

13. Boots C, Stephenson MD. Does obesity increase the risk of miscarriage in spontaneous conception: a systematic review. Semin Reprod Med. 2011;29(6):507–13. doi:10.1055/s-0031-1293204.

14. Metwally M, Saravelos SH, Ledger WL, Li TC. Body mass index and risk of miscarriage in women with recurrent miscarriage. Fertil Steril. 2010;94(1):290–5. doi:10.1016/j.fertnstert.2009.03.021.

15. Lim CC, Mahmood T. Obesity in pregnancy. Best Pract Res Clin Obstet Gynaecol. 2015;29(3):309–19. doi:10.1016/j. bpobgyn.2014.10.008.

16. Anderson JL, Waller DK, Canfield MA, Shaw GM, Watkins ML, Werler MM. Maternal obesity, gestational diabetes, and central nervous system birth defects. Epidemiology. 2005;16(1):87–92.

17. Hendler I, Blackwell SC, Bujold E, Treadwell MC, Mittal P, Sokol RJ, Sorokin Y. Suboptimal second-trimester ultrasonographic visualization of the fetal heart in obese women: should we repeat the examination? J Ultrasound Med. 2005;24(9):1205–9.

18. Mathiesen ER, Ringholm L, Damm P. Stillbirth in diabetic pregnancies. Best Pract Res Clin Obstet Gynaecol. 2011;25(1):105–11. doi:10.1016/j.bpobgyn.2010.11.001.

19. Carlson NS, Hernandez TL, Hurt KJ. Parturition dysfunction in obesity: time to target the pathobiology. Reprod Biol Endocrinol. 2015;13:135. doi:10.1186/s12958-015-0129-6.

20. Kominiarek MA, Zhang J, Vanveldhuisen P, Troendle J, Beaver J, Hibbard JU. Contemporary labor patterns: the impact of maternal body mass index. Am J Obstet Gynecol. 2011;205(3):244 e1–8. doi:10.1016/j.ajog.2011.06.014.

21. Vahratian A, Zhang J, Troendle JF, Savitz DA, Siega-Riz AM. Maternal prepregnancy overweight and obesity and the pattern of labor progression in term nulliparous women. Obstet Gynecol. 2004;104(5 Pt 1):943–51. doi:10.1097/01. AOG.0000142713.53197.91.

22. Dietz PM, Callaghan WM, Morrow B, Cogswell ME. Population-based assessment of the risk of primary cesarean delivery due to excess prepregnancy weight among nulliparous women delivering term infants. Matern Child Health J. 2005;9(3):237–44. doi:10.1007/s10995-005-0003-9.

23. Smid MC, Kearney MS, Stamilio DM. Extreme obesity and post-cesarean wound complications in the Maternal-Fetal Medicine Unit Cesarean Registry. Am J Perinatol. 2015;32(14):1336–41. doi:10.1055/s-0035-1564883.

24. Smid MC, Vladutiu CJ, Dotters-Katz SK, Boggess KA, Manuck TA, Stamilio DM. Maternal obesity and major intraoperative complications during cesarean delivery. Am J Obstet Gynecol. 2017; doi:10.1016/j.ajog.2017.02.011.

25. Smid MC, Dotters-Katz SK, Vaught AJ, Vladutiu CJ, Boggess KA, Stamilio DM. Maternal super obesity and risk for intensive care unit admission in the MFMU cesarean registry. Acta Obstet Gynecol Scand. 2017; doi:10.1111/aogs.13145.

26. Vaananen AJ, Kainu JP, Eriksson H, Lang M, Tekay A, Sarvela J. Does obesity complicate regional anesthesia and result in longer decision to delivery time for emergency cesarean section? Acta Anaesthesiol Scand. 2017;61(6):609–18. doi:10.1111/aas.12891.

27. Aly H, Hammad T, Nada A, Mohamed M, Bathgate S, El-Mohandes A. Maternal obesity, associated complications and risk of prematurity. J Perinatol. 2010;30(7):447–51. doi:10.1038/jp.2009.117.

28. Denison FC, Price J, Graham C, Wild S, Liston WA. Maternal obesity, length of gestation, risk of postdates pregnancy and spontaneous onset of labour at term. BJOG. 2008;115(6):720–5. doi:10.1111/j.1471-0528.2008.01694.x.

29. Carreau AM, Nadeau M, Marceau S, Marceau P, Weisnagel SJ. Pregnancy after bariatric surgery: balancing risks and benefits. Can J Diabetes. 2017; doi:10.1016/j.jcjd.2016.09.005.

30. Yi XY, Li QF, Zhang J, Wang ZH. A meta-analysis of maternal and fetal outcomes of pregnancy after bariatric surgery. Int J Gynaecol Obstet. 2015;130(1):3–9. doi:10.1016/j.ijgo.2015.01.011.

31. Johansson K, Cnattingius S, Naslund I, Roos N, Trolle Lagerros Y, Granath F, Stephansson O, Neovius M. Outcomes of pregnancy after bariatric surgery. N Engl J Med. 2015;372(9):814–24. doi:10.1056/NEJMoa1405789.

32. Simmons D. Diabetes and obesity in pregnancy. Best Pract Res Clin Obstet Gynaecol. 2011;25(1):25–36. doi:10.1016/j.bpobgyn.2010.10.006.

33. American College of Obstetricians and Gynecologists. ACOG Committee opinion no. 548: weight gain during pregnancy. Obstet Gynecol. 2013;121(1):210–2. doi:10.1097/01.AOG.0000425668.87506.4c.

Index

© Springer International Publishing AG 2018
L.E. Moore (ed.), *Diabetes in Pregnancy*,
https://doi.org/10.1007/978-3-319-65518-5

Printed by Printforce, the Netherlands